Ciclosporin in Pediatric Renal Transplantation

CLINICAL RESEARCH SERIES

The aim of this series is to draw attention to results of clinical research projects of interest to physicians in the field of internal medicine and related disciplines.
The editors hope that by reaching a wide audience, it will increase and facilitate practical application of recent findings.

Ciclosporin in Pediatric Renal Transplantation

Proceedings of a Workshop
Scheveningen, December 1985
The Netherlands

Editors:
E.D. Wolff
A.P. Provoost

1986
FORIS PUBLICATIONS
Dordrecht-Holland/Providence-U.S.A.

Published by:
Foris Publications Holland
P.O. Box 509
3300 AM Dordrecht, The Netherlands

Sole distributor for the U.S.A. and Canada:
Foris Publications USA, Inc.
P.O. Box 5904
Providence RI 02903
U.S.A.

ISBN 90 6765 282 2

Printed in the Netherlands by ICG Printing Dordrecht.

Organizing committee:
E.D. Wolff
A.P. Provoost
J. Nauta
J.H.L.J. Bergmeijer

Chairman of the Workshop:
G.B. Haycock

Financial support to the organization of the workshop was given by Sandoz B.V., Nederland.

Ciclosporin in Pediatric Renal Transplantation, E.D. Wolff and A.P. Provoost (editors)

CONTENTS

PREFACE

On December 21st, 1985 a workshop on the use of 'Ciclosporin in Pediatric Renal Transplantation' was held in Scheveningen, The Netherlands. Recently acquired knowledge and views could freely be exchanged by those involved in the use of ciclosporin in pediatric renal transplantation. This volume contains the experiences, results, and opinions from many centers, presented at the workshop.

Ciclosporin has been rapidly introduced into the field of renal transplantation after the experimental and clinical demonstration of its potent immunosuppressive properties. The centers involved in pediatric renal transplantation realised that ciclosporin could have special advantages for children. Through a reduction or the total abandoning of the use of steroids, statural growth of the patients would no longer be hampered. In this way the use of ciclosporin could result in a major breakthrough compared to immunosuppressive regimens incorporating azathioprine and prednisone. The use of ciclosporin in children, however, could bring new problems and unsolved questions. All centers have made their best choice between optimal immunosuppression and minimal ciclosporin associated toxicity. The fact that such a choice is difficult, is evident from the variety of immunosuppressive regimens incorporating the use of ciclosporin.

The workshop was organised by the Departments of Pediatrics (Division of Pediatric Nephrology) and Pediatric Surgery of the Erasmus University and the Sophia Children's Hospital, Rotterdam, The Netherlands, and chaired by G.B. Haycock. The committee has worked enthusiastically to organise the international workshop. We realise that this workshop was only possible thanks to the generous support of Sandoz Nederland BV and the help of the secretarial staff of the Sophia Children's Hospital, Rotterdam as well as many others.

During the workshop a call was voiced to organise a coordinated international study upon the clinical use of ciclosporin in pediatric renal transplantation. The goal of such a study would be to obtain, more efficiently, the clinically relevant data to draw statistically significant conclusions about the optimal use of ciclosporin in children. Many of the participants reacted approvingly of such a plan and we will proceed in order to realise such a study.

It is our hope that the publication of the various contributions to the workshop will stimulate the reader to discussions with the authors and thus may lead to a further optimalisation of the therapeutic management of children receiving a kidney transplant.

Rotterdam, September 1986
E.D. Wolff and A.P. Provoost

TEN YEARS' EXPERIENCE WITH LOW DOSE ALTERNATE DAY PREDNISONE TREATMENT AFTER RENAL TRANSPLANTATION IN CHILDREN

J. NAUTA[1], A.J. VAN DER HEIJDEN[1], N.J. LANGENDOEN[1], D.L. WESTBROEK[2], J. JEEKEL[2], J.H.L.J. BERGMEIJER[3], J.C. MOLENAAR[3], and E.D. WOLFF[1]

[1]*Department of Pediatrics, Division of Nephrology,* [2]*Department of General Surgery and* [3]*Department of Pediatric Surgery*
Sophia Children's Hospital and Erasmus University Medical School, Rotterdam, The Netherlands

During a ten year period, 46 children received 53 renal transplantations and were managed successfully with a standard immunosuppressive regimen using AZA in combination with a long-term schedule of low doses of Prednisone administered on alternate days. A high, once daily dose was given initially, generally not exceeding 3 months after transplantation. Overall graft survival was good, amounting to 68% five years after transplantation. Major causes of graft failure were acute thrombosis in four, acute rejection in four and chronic rejection in seven cases. Forty-four of 46 patients are currently alive. Patient growth was relatively good. Anti-hypertensive medication was required in only 15% of the patients two years after transplantation. Aseptic bone necrosis occurred in two patients, while cataracts were noted in 17% of the patients. The lowe dose schedule for Prednisone administration resembles that employed in most centres that have reverted to CyA and as such our regimen using AZA and Prednisone may serve as a basis for the evaluation of modern immunosuppression.

Renal transplantation has generally been accepted as the ultimate treatment for children with end-stage renal disease [1]. Many complications presenting after transplantation are related to the immunosuppressive therapy. In 1976, Borel [2] discovered the immunosuppressive effect of Ciclosporin (CyA), which led to Calne [3] putting this to clinical use. Since then CyA is increasingly reported as a major advance in immunosuppression improving its effectiveness and reducing side effects of corticosteroids, resulting from a decreased use of Prednisone [4–7]. However, the incidence of such side effects varied widely between centres, depending on divergent Prednisone dosage schedules in conventional immunosuppression. In our renal transplantation programme we employed a conventional immunosuppressive regimen with Azathioprine (AZA), but our long-term dosage schedule for Prednisone was comparable to that used in modern regimens. Our ten year's experience with this regimen may provide a valuable basis for evaluating modern immunosuppression.

Correspondence to: J. Nauta, Nephrology division, Sophia Children's Hospital, Gordelweg 160, 3038 GE Rotterdam, The Netherlands

PATIENTS AND METHODS

The programme for dialysis and transplantation at the Sophia Children's Hospital in Rotterdam was started in August 1974. Between then and July 1985, 60 children out of a regional population of 2.5 million, entered into the programme. The type and frequency of primary renal disease in these children is shown in figure 1. Compared with other pediatric centres, there was a relatively high frequency of obstructive uropathy and haemolytic uremic syndrome, both involving boys only, which explains an overall male to female ratio of 2:1. Excluded from the programme were children with incurable cancer, severe mental retardation, or advanced metabolic disease.

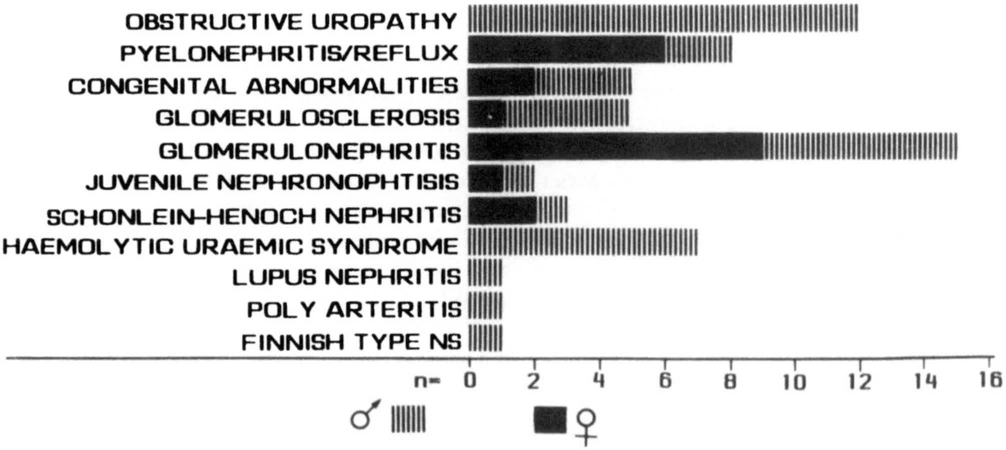

Fig.1 Primary renal disease (n=60).

All patients were on dialysis, 54 hemodialysis versus 6 peritoneal, until a suitable donor kidney became available. The average waiting time was 10 months. Seven patients died during that time. The first transplantation was carried out in July 1975 and by July 1985 a total of 46 children had received an allograft, seven of them twice, amounting to 53 transplantations altogether. The age of the children at the time of transplantation varied from 6.3 to 17.9 years.

The kidneys were all obtained from cadaver donors and matched for HLA antigens according to the standard Eurotransplant matching programme [8]. On average, there were 1.4 mismatches for the HLA-A and B loci (n = 53) and 0.6 mismatches for the HLA-Dr locus (n = 33). The first warm ischemic time averaged 4 minutes (range 0–20) while the average for the second warm ischemic time was 41 minutes (range 21–75). Average cold ischemic time amounted to 25 hours (range 12–40). Donor age varied from 2 to 46 years, with 50% under 18 years of age. Four donors were less than 5 years old.

Immunosuppressive regimen

Before transplantation, each patient had at least one blood transfusion, with the total number ranging from 1 to 50 per patient. AZA was started a few hours before transplantation and continued indefinitely in a single morning dose of 3 mg/kg body weight. The dose was reduced when lymphocytopenia developed. There was generally no adjustment of dosage for growth. Prednisone (or methylprednisolone) was started after transplantation, for the first two weeks also in a single morning dose of 3 mg/kg body weight. After that the dose was gradually reduced to 30 mg each morning, regardless of body weight, to be replaced with alternate day administration of 60 mg in a single morning dose, generally within three months after transplantation. Subsequently, the dose was reduced by 5 mg approximately every two weeks, until a maintenance dose was achieved of 10–20 mg every 48 hours, usually within six months after transplantation. On day 0, 3, 7, 14, and 21, the recipients received a morning dose of 10 mg/kg body weight methylprednisolone. Rejection episodes were treated with additional methylprednisolone on alternate days in a morning dose of 20 mg/kg for six to ten days. We never used antithymocyte globulin, while plasmapheresis was only carried out in two patients with acute rejection symptoms unresponsive to standard rejection therapy.

Surgical procedure

The native kidneys were only removed on medical indication, for example in case of severe hypertension or infection. None of the patients underwent splenectomy. All donor kidneys were transplanted retroperitoneally into the iliac fossa. Vessel anastomoses were constructed end-to-end or end-to-side, depending on anatomical relations. Capsulotomy was performed routinely and a biopsy was taken 30 minutes after reperfusion. All donor ureters were implanted into the bladder. An anti-reflux procedure was introduced in 1979 for the ureter-bladder anastomosis.

The fluid balance was corrected pre-operatively, aimed at a well-hydrated state without clinical evidence of fluid overload. During the arterial anastomosis, all patients received Mannitol (2 g/kg BW maximally 50 g) and Furosemide (2 mg/kg BW). Post-operatively, the fluid balance was carefully maintained, including correction for losses into the tissues. Optimal central and periferal circulation was maintained by controlling the clinical parameters without intra-arterial or central venous pressure measurements. Post-operative treatment also included barrier nursing, administration of antibiotics and bladder catheterisation during the first two weeks.

RESULTS

Forty-four of the 46 patients who received renal allografts during the 10 years study period, have survived up till now. One patient died 33 months after transplantation because a nonresectable fibroma or fibrosarcoma had developed in the transplant area concomitant to recurrent focal segmental glomerulosclerosis. This patient had undergone a 6 months course of cyclophosphamide before entering the programme. A second child died after 11 months following a cerebrovascular accident, probably secondary to thrombosis. Thirty of the 46 patients are doing well after one transplantation and so are four of the seven patients that received a second allograft. Figure 2 is a schematic presentation of the patients and their treatment modalities.

The graft survival rate was 81% after the first year, dropping to 68% five years after transplantation. Figure 3 shows the actuarial graft survival rate for all transplantations during the first five years. In the first three months of the programme, we lost as many grafts as during the following five years. There were 17 cases

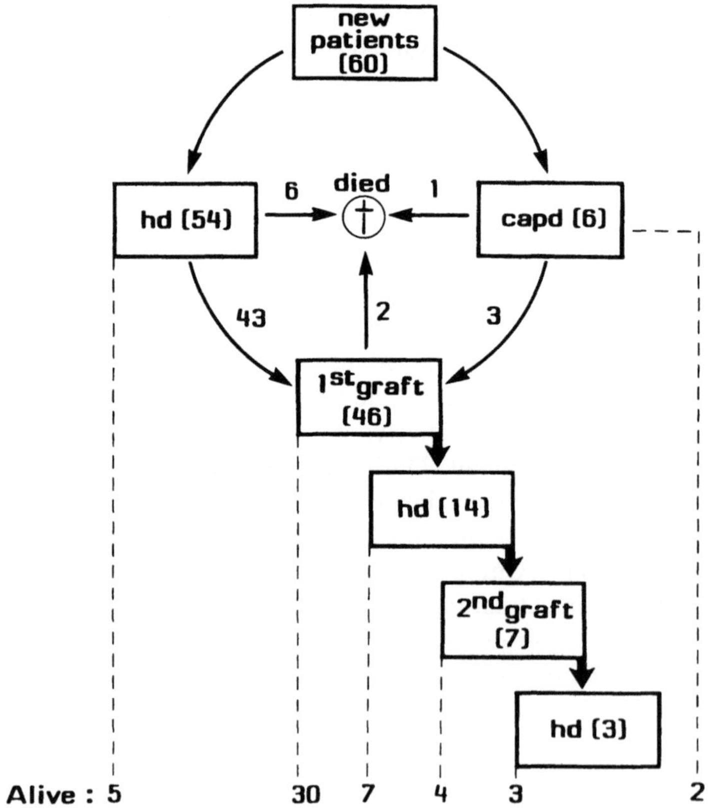

Fig.2 The patients and their treatment modalities.

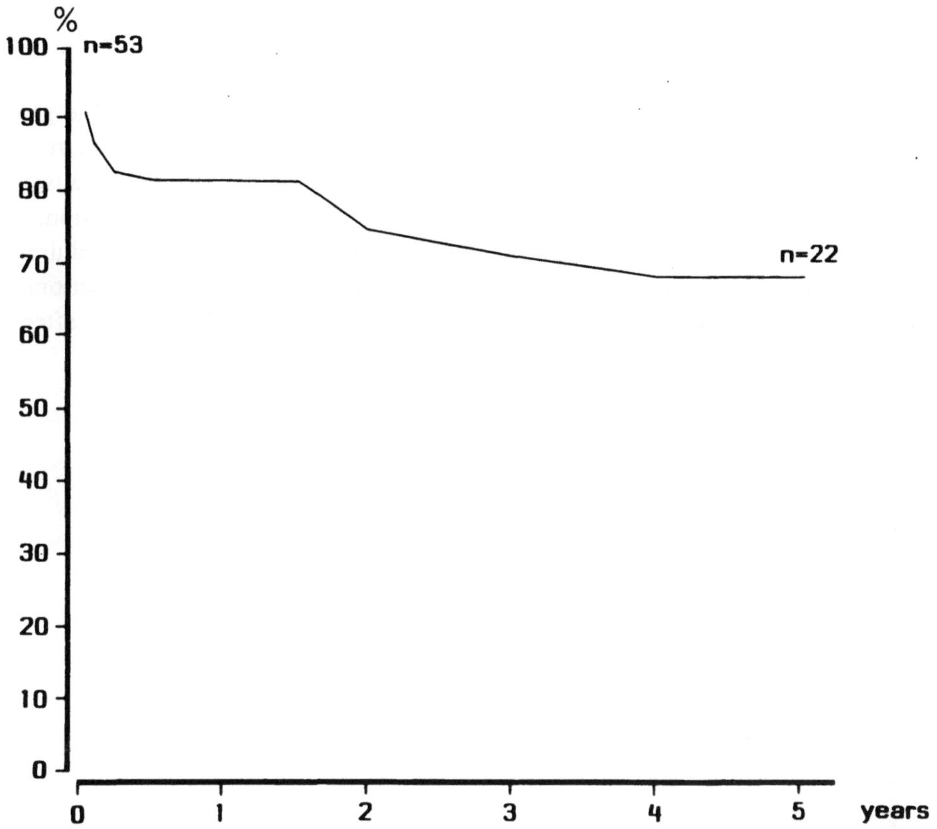

**Fig.3 Actuarial graft survival.
First and second cadavergrafts combined.**

of graft failure altogether, three times involving a second graft. All three grafts with donorage under three years of age failed within one year after transplantation. Table I lists the causes of graft failure. In four cases this was acute thrombosis,

TABLE I

Cause of graft failure

n	cause of failure	function duration	
4	thrombosis	0,1,2,6*	wks
2	acute rejection	4,10	wks
1	storage failure	6	wks
2	RAS	10,16*	wks
1	necrotic ureter	6	wks
7	chronic rejection	$1^1/_2$,2,2,2,$3^1/_2$,$5^1/_2$,$8^1/_2$	yrs

*associated with acute rejection

without clinical or histological evidence of rejection in three of them. The fourth case was associated with acute rejection which also occurred in one of the two cases of renal artery stenosis. Acute rejection was the direct or indirect cause of four graft losses altogether, from 4 to 16 weeks after transplantation. One graft was lost due to bacterial infection of ischaemic laesions already present at transplantation ('storage failure'). Chronic rejection was the major, long-term cause of graft failure, occurring in seven cases from 1.5 to 8.5 years after transplantation.

Within two days after transplantation, 83% of the grafts had achieved a diuresis of more than one litre per day. The mean plasma creatinine of the functioning grafts gradually increased from 95 μmol/1 after 3 weeks to 158 μmol/1 after 5 years (see figure 4).

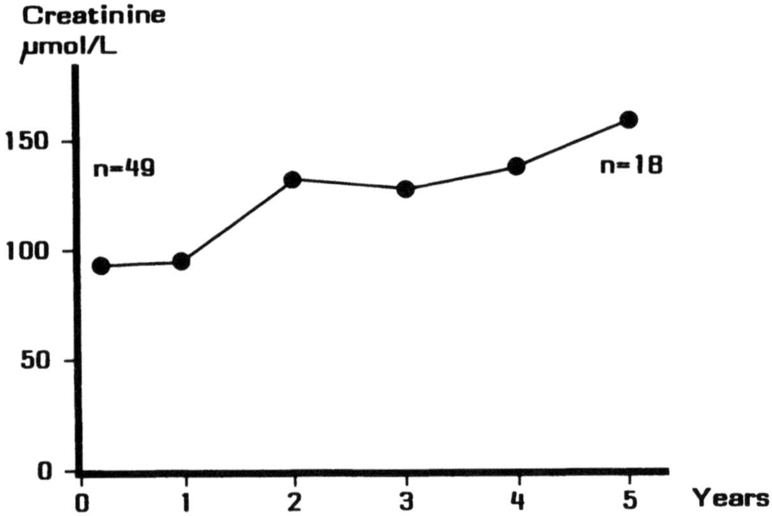

Fig.4 Mean plasma creatinine of functioning grafts.

Patient growth was evaluated in 30 patients with a mean age of 12 years and a mean height of –2.5 SD at transplantation. The mean follow-up for these patients was 4.5 years, with a minimum of one year. Growth is expressed as the average annual change in the standard deviation score for height (SDS/yr). Average growth was reasonable, without a significant change in SDS (–0.06 SDS/yr); 14 patients improved their SDS, while 16 did not. In 21 patients with reasonable renal function (plasma creatinine < 150 μmol/1) and a boy:girl ratio of 13:8, we noted normal growth in the boys (–0.02 SDS/yr) and slightly increased growth in the girls (+0.20 SDS/yr). Comparing the prepubertal children (boys < 11 yrs, girls < 9 yrs) with the older ones, growth was not better for the 11 prepubertal children (–0.09 SDS/yr).

No patients were lost due to infectious complications. Bacterial infections included

10 urinary tract infections and 3 respiratory tract infections. One graft was lost after infection of large ischaemic laesions, already noted at transplantation. Viral infections with clinical symptoms were caused by herpes in two cases, and in one case each by cytomegalovirus, varicella zoster, and mumps.

A Cushingoid appearance was noted in most patients. This proved to be reversible in all of them within the first six months after transplantation. Half the number of recipients required anti-hypertensive medication during the first half year after transplantation, but only 15% of all patients needed anti-hypertensive treatment for more than two years. Aseptic necrosis of the bone, involving the femoral head, was seen in two patients. Routine ophtalmic examination twice a year revealed a posttransplantation development of cataracts in 17% of the patients. This was always of a minor degree.

DISCUSSION

Compared with conventional immunosuppressive regimens used in other pediatric centres, we administered relatively high doses of corticosteroids during the first three months after transplantation. However, all immunosuppressive drugs were consistently given in single morning doses, while an early changeover to an alternate day schedule following gradual but drastic reduction of dosage was also aimed at minimising the risk of side effects. Modern immunosuppressive regimens using CyA also employ low dosage schemes for Prednisone. As such, our conventional regimen could provide a basis for the clinical evaluation of modern immunosuppression.

Our patient and graft survival rate are relatively good [9–13]. In the two patients that died, the cause of death might have been related to the immunosuppressive medication. The development of fibroma or fibrosarcoma in one of them may have been secondary to a combination of standard immunosuppression and a previous, extended course of cyclophosphamide. The occurrence of cerebral thrombosis in the second patient may be explained by the increased risk of thrombosis reportedly associated with the use of corticosteroids [14].

Short-term as well as long-term graft survival was good. More effective immunosuppression during the first months after transplantation, e.g. using CyA, might have prevented the four graft losses directly or indirectly caused by acute rejection. However, in 90% of our transplantations there was little indication that CyA would have improved the results regarding graft survival or graft function. Acute thrombosis of the allograft, apart from or associated with rejection, was a major cause of graft failure. While the high initial dosage of corticosteroids might have been a contributive factor in the frequency of renal vascular thrombosis, it is by no means certain that this frequency would have been lower if CyA had been used [7, 15, 16]. Chronic rejection was the major cause of long-term graft failure and consequently it is to be hoped that more advanced immunosuppressive medication may provide more effective prevention of this type of rejection in the future. As our series was relatively small, graft failure could not be associated with HLA-matching, duration of ischaemic time, donor age, number of previous transplants, or number of previous blood transfusions.

On the whole there was a relatively low frequency of long-term side effects of corticosteroids. Patient growth was reasonable and in agreement with the data reported by other centres employing alternate day Prednisone schedules [17]. Here again, our series was too small to draw a definite conclusion.

Infection was a common post-operative complication in our patients, although this was never fatal and only one graft was lost because of infection. Aseptic necrosis of the bone developed in 2 of our 46 patients, comparing favourably with other reports ranging from 3–41% [18]. We also had a relatively low frequency of cataracts (17%) compared with other reports ranging from 14–83% [19].

In conclusion, our early changeover to a low dose, alternate day schedule for Prednisone administration in combination with AZA, has resulted in adequate immunosuppression with a relatively low frequency of steroid side effects in pediatric renal transplantation. In view of the similarity in schedule for Prednisone administration, this standard immunosuppressive regimen may serve to evaluate modern immunosuppressive regimens using CyA.

ACKNOWLEDGMENT

The authors are indepted to Mrs A.M.C. Ribbink-Goslinga for linguistic advice.

REFERENCES

1 Novello A.C., Fine R.N. Renal transplantation in children. A review. Int. J. Pediatr. Nephrol. 1982; 3:87–98.

2 Borel J.F., Feurer C., Gubler H.U., Stähelin H. Biological effects of Cyclosporin A: a new antilymphocytic agent. Agents Actions 1976; 6:468–475.

3 Calne R.Y., White D.J.G., Thiru S., Evans D.B., Mc. Master P., Dunn, D.C., Craddock G.N., Pentlow B.D., Rolles K. Cyclosporin A in patients receiving renal allografts from cadaver donors. Lancet 1978; ii:1323–1327.

4 Ferguson R.M., Rynasiewicz J.J., Sutherland D.E.R., Simmons R.L., Najarian J.S. Cyclosporin A in renal transplantation: a prospective randomized trial. Surgery 1982; 92:175–181.

5 The Canadian Multicentre Transplant Study Group. A randomized clinical trial of Cyclosporine in cadaveric renal transplantation. N. Engl. J. Med. 1983; 309:809–815.

6 Merion R.M., White D.J., Thiru S., Evans D.B., Calne R.Y. Cyclosporine: five years' experience in cadaveric renal transplantation. N. Engl. J. Med. 1984; 310:148–154.

7 Wolff E.D., Provoost A.P. (eds). Ciclosporin in pediatric renal transplantation. Foris Publications 1986.

8 Persijn G.G. HLA-matching and blood transfusion(s) in renal transplantation. Doctoral Thesis State University Leiden, 1985.

9 Chantler C., Carter J.E., Bewick M., Counahan R., Cameron J.S., Ogg, C.S., Williams G., Winder E. Ten year's experience with regular hemodialysis and renal transplantation. Arch. Dis. Child. 1980; 55:435–445.

10 Arbus G.S., Galiwango J., De Maria J.E., Churchill B.M., Irwin M.A. The first 10 years of the dialysis-transplantation program at the Hospital for Sick Children, Toronto. 2: Transplantation and complications of chronic renal failure. Can. Med. Assoc. J. 1980; 120:659–664.

11 Fine R.M., Malekzadeh M.H., Pennisi A.J., Ettenger R.B., Uittenbogaart C.H., Negrete V.F., Korsch B.M. Long-term results of renal transplantation in children. Pediatrics 1978; 61:641–650.

12 Potter D.E., Holliday M.A., Piel C.F., Feduska N.J., Belzer F.O., Salvatierra O. Treatment of end-stage renal disease in children: a 15-year experience. Kidney Int. 1980; 18:103–109.

13 Broyer M., Gagnadoux M.F., Guest G., Busson M., Beurton D. Résultats de 310 transplantations de rein de cadavre chez l'enfant et l'adolescent. Arch. Fr. Pediatr. 1985; 42:237–243.

14 Dukes M.N.G. ed. Meyler's side effects of drugs: an encyclopaedia of adverse reactions and interactions. 9th ed. Amsterdam: Excerpta Medica, 1980; 650 pp.

15 Vanrenterghem Y., Lerut T., Roels L., Gruwez J., Michielsen P., Gresele P., Colucci M., Deckmyn H., Arnout J., Vermylen J. Thromboembolic complications and haemostatic changes in Cyclosporin-treated cadaveric kidney allograft recipients. Lancet 1985; i:999–1002.

16 Neild G.H., Reuben R., Hartley R.B., Cameron J.S. Glomerular thrombi in renal allografts associated with cyclosporin treatment. J. Clin. Pathol. 1985; 38:253–258.

17 Bosque M., Munian A., Bewick M., Haycock G., Chantler C. Growth after renal transplants. Arch. Dis. Child. 1983; 58:110–114.

18 Van Boven W.P.L. Aseptic necrosis of bone following a successful kidney transplantation. Doctoral Thesis State University Groningen, 1980.

19 Polak B.C.P. Ophtalmological complications of haemodialysis and kidney transplantation: with special note on hereditary renal diseases. Doctoral Thesis State University Leiden, 1980.

REVERSIBILITY OF CICLOSPORIN RELATED SIDE EFFECTS IN ADULT RECIPIENTS AFTER ONE YEAR OF CONTINUOUS THERAPY

D.J. VERSLUIS, G.J. WENTING, F.H.M. DERKX, M.A.D.H. SCHALEKAMP, J. JEEKEL and W. WEIMAR

Departments of Internal Medicine I and General Surgery, University Hospital Rotterdam-Dijkzigt, Rotterdam, The Netherlands

In the mid seventies the new immunosuppressant ciclosporin (CyA) was isolated from the cultures of the soil fungus Tolypocladium Inflatum Gams. Initial experiments showed its selective inhibition of T-cell activity. Further animal studies reveiled that CyA acts by inhibiting lymfokine mediated T-helper functions, required for B-cell activation, cytotoxic T-cell generation and proliferation of T-cell subpopulations. Because of its potency in the prevention of organ allograft rejection and the absence of side effects in laboratory animal experiments, CyA was soon introduced in clinical transplantation. At our centre the one year graft survival after renal transplantation in adult patients showed a significant improvement from 70% under azathioprine (AZA) therapy to 80% after the introduction of CyA, while the incidence of acute rejection episodes decreased from 88% to 35%. However, CyA therapy is accompanied by unwanted side effects [1]. Nephrotoxicity and hypertension are the most frequent and clinically important complications, as at least 50% of renal allograft recipients under CyA medication show impaired renal function and a persistent elevation of blood pressure, requiring antihypertensive therapy. Because CyA nephrotoxicity seemed to be partly reversible after dose reduction it was hoped that no serious kidney damage would develop during long term CyA treatment. However, recently it has been suggested that prolonged CyA therapy may lead to irreversible and progressive nephropathy, involving structural renal damage [2]. Myers et al. (from the Stanford heart transplantation group) reported serious renal dysfunction in 17 of 32 heart transplant recipients treated with CyA for more than one year, including two patients who ultimately required dialysis therapy for end stage renal failure. To avoid these long term sequelae, switching the immunosuppressive regimen from CyA to AZA has been suggested. Several studies were concerned with this conversion of therapy which was performed at fixed intervals three or six months after kidney transplantation [3–6]. In all studies an improvement in serum creatinine has been found. However, these early

Correspondence to: W. Weimar, Department of Internal Medicine I, University Hospital Rotterdam-Dijkzigt, Dr. Molewaterplein 40, 3015 GD Rotterdam, The Netherlands.

conversions resulted in a high incidence of acute allograft rejection (approximately 30%), some of which proved to be irreversible. We continued CyA therapy in our adult transplant recipients for one year in an attempt to induce a safer engraftment. At that time we were able to study in detail the potential reversibility of chronic CyA related nephrotoxicity and hypertension.

PATIENTS AND METHODS

In the period November 1983–August 1984, 41 consecutive non-diabetic adult patients received a cadaveric renal allograft. CyA was started six hours after transplantation at a dose of 4 mg/kg/day given by continuous infusion for the first 36–48 hours. The initial oral dosage was 14 mg/kg/day given in 2 divided doses. CyA plasma trough levels were kept between 50–150 ng/ml. CyA plasma levels were measured using the commercially available radio-immunoassay kit (Sandoz Ltd, Basle, Switzerland). Prednisone (15 mg/day) was given from the day of transplantation. Episodes of acute rejection were confirmed by percutaneous allograft biopsies. Therapy for rejection consisted of a 21 day course of rabbit anti-thymocyte globulin (RIV, Bilthoven, the Netherlands) given in a dose of 4 mg/kg at varying intervals to keep the number of circulating T-cells between 50–150/mm^3. The all-over actuarial one year graft survival was 81% and the one year patient survival 95%. In ten of the 33 recipients with a functioning graft one year after transplantation, immunosuppressive therapy had already been changed to AZA before the year was over, mainly to distinguish rejection from CyA nephrotoxicity. Our study group consisted of the remaining 23 patients who had received one year of continuous CyA therapy. All patients had a stable kidney function and had not experienced a rejection episode in the 6 months before admission to our metabolic ward. Patients received a diet with a fixed sodium content (40–50 mmol/day). We measured effective renal plasma flow (ERPF) by the clearance of ^{131}I-sodium-iodo-hippurate. The radio label was administered by a constant infusion following a loading dose. Serum levels were obtained at three thirty minutes intervals after an equilibration period of ninety minutes. In calculating the clearance mean values were used. Blood pressure was recorded by an automatic device at five minutes intervals during an hour. Plasma renin activity was measured by radio-immunoassay. Fasting blood samples were taken to determine cholesterol and triglycerides after which a 75 gram oral glucose tolerance test was performed. At the last day of admission CyA was stopped and AZA was started in a dose of 2 mg/kg/day. Three months after conversion the patients were readmitted to our ward for a similar second evaluation. Statistical analysis was performed using Chi-square test and the Student's t-test for paired data.

RESULTS

Acute rejection

Within 6 weeks after conversion a biopsy proven rejection was diagnosed in 5 of the 23 patients (22%). Rejection episodes were significantly more frequent in recipients of a second allograft ($p < 0.01$) (Table I). Four of the seven (57%) recipients of a second allograft showed acute rejection and two of them eventually lost their graft. One out of the 16 (6%) patients who received a first kidney also showed rejection. Rejecting patients did not differ significantly from non-rejecting patients in respect of preconversion renal function, the number of preconversion rejection episodes, CyA trough levels or HLA-matching. After the initial six weeks after conversion no further rejection episodes were diagnosed during a follow-up period of 6–18 months. One patient showed a recurrence of a membrano-proliferative glomerulonephritis within 3 months after conversion.

TABLE I

Preconversion characteristics of patients with and without rejection after conversion

	No rejection	Rejection
Number of Patients	18	5
First/second transplants	15/3	1/4*
Number of mismatches HLA-AB	1.50 ± 0.25	2.20 ± 0.6
HLA-DR	0.61 ± 0.12	0.60 ± 0.4
Lymphocytotoxic antibodies (%)	29 ± 7	44 ± 8**
Mean number of rejection episodes before conversion	0.3	0.4
CyA dose (mg/kg/day)	6.4 ± 1.1	5.2 ± 0.8
CyA trough levels (ng/ml)	106 ± 16	69 ± 8
Creatinine clearance (ml/min)	46 ± 3	57 ± 7

* $p < 0.01$ Chi-square test
** $p < 0.01$ Student's t-test

Renal function and blood pressure

The remaining 17 transplant recipients were studied as described before. Serum creatinine dropped from 171 ± 12 μmol/l to 129 ± 7 μmol/l (mean ± SEM) at 3 months after conversion ($p < 0.01$). This decline of 25% was already reached at 3 weeks after conversion and remained stable afterwards. Creatinine clearance showed an increase from 47 ± 3 ml/min to 66 ± 4 ml/min at the second study period ($p < 0.01$), which is an improvement of 40% in glomerular filtration rate (fig. I). ERPF rose from 211 ± 11 to 255 ± 14 ml/min ($p < 0.01$) after conversion

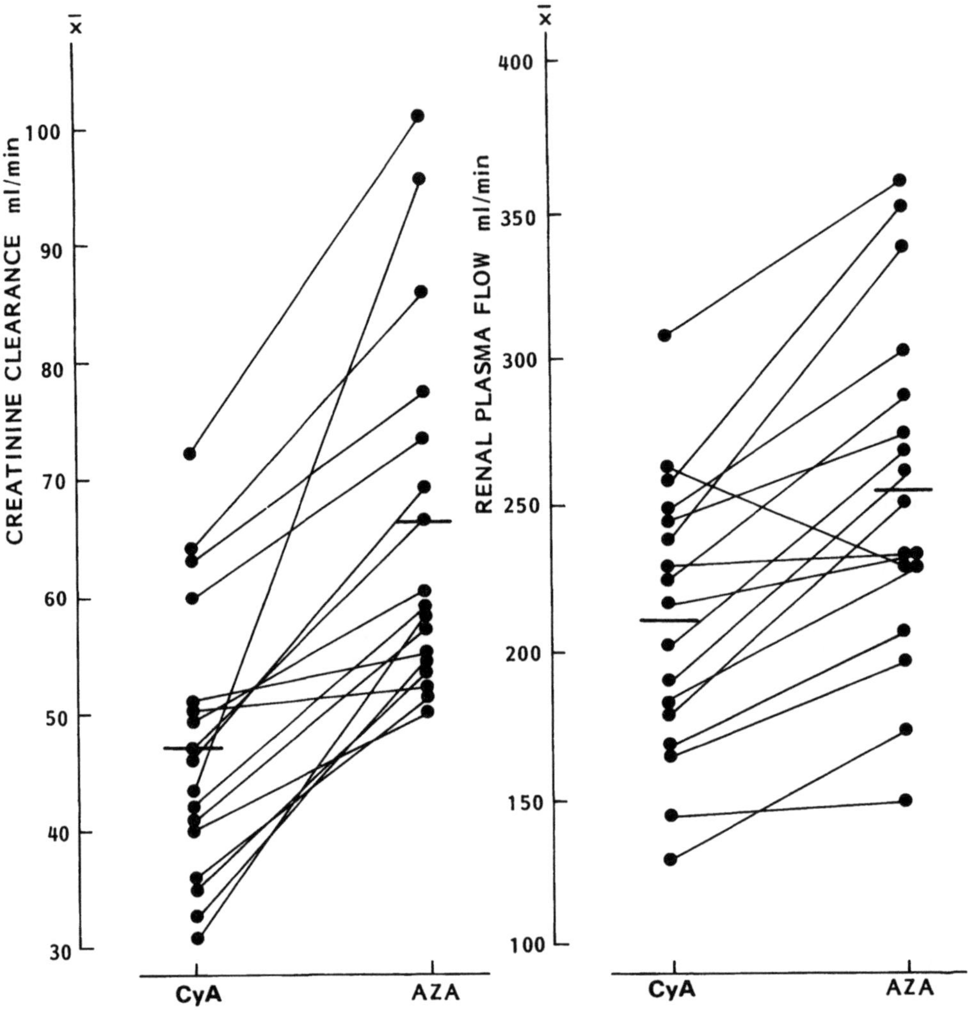

Fig. 1. Effect of conversion from CyA to AZA on creatinine clearance and effective renal plasma flow at 3 months after conversion.

(21%). Before conversion 12/17 patients received antihypertensive treatment, which was continued during our study. After stopping CyA therapy blood pressure decreased from 142/90 to 123/77 mmHg without a change in heart rate ($p < 0.01$). Plasma renin activity showed a rise from 15.2 to 25.1 μU/ml ($p < 0.01$).

Metabolic side effects

After conversion fasting glucose levels did not change (4.5 ± 0.2 vs 4.3 ± 0.1 mmol/1), but a significant fall in 2 hour glucose levels after oral glucose tolerance test was found (7.2 ± 0.5 vs 5.5 ± 0.3 mmol/1, $p < 0.05$ (Table II). We also

TABLE II

Metabolic indices before and three months after conversion (n= 17) mean ± SEM

	CyA	AZA
Serum cholesterol (mmol/l)	8.0 ± 0.5	6.5 ± 0.4 *
Serum triglycerides (mmol/l)	3.2 ± 0.3	2.2 ± 0.2 *
Serum glucose before loading (mmol/l)	4.5 ± 0.2	4.3 ± 0.1
Serum glucose 2 hrs after loading (mmol/l)	7.2 ± 0.5	5.5 ± 0.5**

* $p < 0.01$ Student's t-test
** $p < 0.05$ Student's t-test

found a significant reduction in serum cholesterol (8.0 ± 0.5 to 6.5 ± 0.4 mmol/l, $p < 0.01$) and serum triglycerides (3.2 ± 0.3 to 2.2 ± 0.2 mmol/l, $p < 0.01$). The decreases in cholesterol and triglycerides were not correlated with an improvement in any of the renal function indices (Spearman–Rank test).

DISCUSSION

In the present study the continuation of CyA therapy for one year after renal transplantation in adults did not result in a safer engraftment than has been reported by other centres, where CyA had been given for shorter episodes. Our overall incidence of post-conversion rejection of 22% is comparable to the results of those studies where conversion was performed at 3 or at 6 months after transplantation [3–6]. However, we were able to predict the risk for post-conversion rejection as the incidence of this complication was 57% in recipients of a second allograft and only 6% in the patients who had received a first kidney. For the latter group conversion from CyA to AZA is a safe procedure and should be performed when the benefits of changing therapy outweigh the risks of long term CyA treatment. One of these risks could be the progressive and irreversible renal damage due to an intrinsic nephrotoxicity of CyA. We found, however, no evidence for this complication one year after CyA therapy. Stopping CyA after one year showed an important improvement of renal function. The rapid decline of serum creatinine, within 3 weeks after conversion, is a strong argument against irreversible kidney damage due to CyA. The outspoken rise in glomerular filtration rate in relation to the increase in ERPF suggests a reversible effect of CyA on the afferent glomerular arteriole. The dramatic decrease in blood pressure after conversion is also remarkable. The lower values of plasma renin activity before conversion compared to those during AZA therapy reflects a low renin hypertension during CyA treatment, which argues against involvement of the renin-angiotensin-aldosterone system in the CyA induced changes in renal hemodynamics. Probably this phenomenon is regulated by other hitherto unknown mechanisms. In accordance with recent observations

[7] we found that conversion to AZA was associated with an improvement in glucose tolerance and a fall in serum cholesterol and triglycerides. This is probably the result of the enhanced clearance of prednisone after stopping CyA [8] as we found no correlation between the improvement in renal function indices and the fall serum lipids. In conclusion, we have shown that even after one year of therapy the CyA related renal dysfunction and hypertension is reversible, which also holds true for the metabolic side effects of CyA. Therefore, we feel that the fear for irreversible structural renal damage or metabolic defects due to long-term CyA therapy is not warranted and cannot be an argument in favour of elective conversion from CyA to AZA. In recipients of a second allograft this procedure is even contraindicated because of the high risk of post conversion rejection. However, in recipients of a first transplant where safe conversion is possible, the sequelae of long term hypertension, elevated serum lipids, impaired glucose tolerance and the high costs of therapy remain arguments in favour of conversion despite the reversibility of these side-effects after stopping CyA. Especially in children these factors should be considered and weighed against the potential beneficial effects of long-term CyA therapy on graft survival.

ACKNOWLEDGEMENTS

We thank Mrs. J. Blazer-v.d. Werken and Mrs. W. Zuidema for secretarial help.

REFERENCES

1 Krupp P., Timonen P., Gülich A. Side effects and safety of Sandimmun in long-term treatment of transplant patients. In: Ciclosporin in autoimmune diseases. Schindler R. (ed.), Springer-Verlag, 1985; pp 43–49.

2 Myers B.D., Ross J., Newton L., Luetscher J., Perlroth M. Cyclosporine-associated chronic nephropathy. N. Engl. J. Med. 1984; 311:699–705.

3 Morris P.J., French M.E., Dunnill M.S., Hunnisett A.G.W., Ting A., Thompson J.F., Wood R.F.M. A controlled trial of Cyclosporine in renal transplantation with conversion to azathioprine and prednisolone after three months. Transplantation 1983; 36:273–277.

4 Chapman J.R., Harding N.G.L., Griffiths D., Morris P.J. Reversibility of Cyclosporin nephrotoxicity after three month's treatment. Lancet 1985; i:128–130.

5 Rocher L.L., Milford E.L., Kirkman R.L., Carpenter C.B., Strom T.B., Tilney N.L. Conversion from Cyclosporine to azathioprine in renal allograft recipients. Transplantation 1984; 38:669–674.

6 Stuart F.P., Haag B.W., Jones K., Stuart J.K., Thistlethwaite J.R. Conversion from Cyclosporine to azathioprine therapy six months after kidney transplantation. Transpl. Proc. 1985; 17:2681–2682.

7 Harris K.P.G., Russell G.I., Veitch P.S., Walls J. Alterations in lipid and carbohydrate metabolism attributable to Cyclosporin A in renal transplant recipients. Br. Med. J. 1986; 292:16

8 Öst L. Effects of Cyclosporin on prednisolone metabolism. Lancet 1984; i:451.

COMPARATIVE CICLOSPORIN NEPHROTOXICITY IN YOUNG AND ADULT RATS WITH A DIMINISHED FUNCTION

ABRAHAM P. PROVOOST

Department of Pediatric Surgery, Erasmus University, Rotterdam, The Netherlands

The effect of CyA was studied in male Wistar rats aged 3 or 13 weeks. Three surgical interventions were used. These included a sham operation (2K), unilateral nephrectomy (NX) and a combination of 45 min of warm ischemia plus contralateral nephrectomy (IS+NX). Vehicle treated rats that underwent the same surgical procedures served as controls. The CyA, in a dose of 15 mg/kg, was administered intramusculary 5 times a week for a period of 4 weeks. The GFR was determined during and after the treatment course.

In adult rats it was noted for all three models that the GFR was less in the CyA treated rats than in the vehicle treated rats during the 4 weeks treatment period. The degree of impairment, however, differed in the various models. At the end of the treatment course, the GFR of the CyA treated rats (expressed as a percentage of the controls) amounted to 84% in 2K rats, 64% in NX rats, and 46% in IS+NX rats. After cessation of the CyA administration, there was a complete recovery of the GFR to control levels in 2K and NX rats. In IS+NX rats the GFR remained significantly below that of controls. We conclude that in adult rats, ischemically damaged kidneys are more vulnerable to the nephrotoxic effects than intact kidneys. In adult rats, CyA seems to interfere with processes such as compensatory hypertrophy and recovery after unilateral nephrectomy or renal ischemia.

In young rats normal development of the GFR was only slightly affected by the CyA treatment. The degree of impairment in the GFR in NX and IS+NX young rats did not differ from that found in young 2K rats. After cessation of the treatment there was a complete recovery in all 3 models. We conclude that in contrast with the effect of CyA on adult rat kidneys, CyA does not interfere with the compensatory hypertrophy or the recovery from ischemia in young developing kidneys.

In 1978, at the first clinical use of ciclosporin (CyA) in renal transplantation, the nephrotoxic side effects of this potent immunosuppressive agent were recognized [1,2]. Up till then the nephrotoxicity of CyA had been demonstrated in animal studies but at much higher doses than required for immunosuppression [3,4]. Unfortunately, the nephrotoxicity of CyA was generally studied in animals with intact kidneys. In renal transplantation, the kidney is in a compromised state and has to show recovery as well as compensatory hypertrophy to reach its final level of renal function. We surmised that the effects of CyA might be more severe when administered in a situation where the kidneys also had to cope with a sudden

Correspondence to: A.P. Provoost, Dept. of Pediatric Surgery, Laboratory for Surgery, Erasmus University, P.O. Box 1738, 3000 DR Rotterdam, The Netherlands impairment in function. Consequently, we studied the effects of CyA upon the glomerular filtration rate (GFR) in adult and young rats in which a functional renal response was induced either by unilateral nephrectomy (NX) or by a combination of a temporary renal ischemia and contralateral nephrectomy (IS+NX). This combination represents a model for renal transplantation in the absence of the complicating effects of rejection.

MATERIALS AND METHODS

Male rats of a Wistar strain (Wistar Cpb/WU, TNO, Zeist, The Netherlands) were used. Adult rats were about 13 weeks old with a body weight (BW) of about 300 grams. Young rats were about 3 weeks old and just weaned with a BW of about 50 grams at the start of the experiments. Food (standard rat chow) and tap water were available ad libitum.

Renal function measurement

The GFR was determined in pentobarbital (60 mg/kg, intraperitoneally) anesthetized rats. The method allowing for repeated use within the same animal has been described in detail elsewhere [5]. The GFR was measured during treatment at 1, 2, and 4 weeks after the first CyA administration as well as 1, 3, and 6 weeks after the cessation of the CyA administration.

Surgery

All interventions were performed under ether anesthesia. For a unilateral nephrectomy the left kidney was approached through a midline incision, the renal pedicle was ligated and the kidney removed. For unilateral ischemia plus contralateral nephrectomy, the right kidney was mobilized and a small bulldog clamp was placed on the right renal artery. After 45 min of ischemia the clamp was removed. Subsequently, the left kidney was removed as described above. The two-kidney control rats (2K) underwent a sham operation. The kidneys were mobilized but otherwise left intact.

Ciclosporin administration

CyA, in a concentration of 100 mg/ml (Sandimmun, Sandoz, Basel), was diluted with olive oil to a concentration of 15 mg/ml. The CyA was administered intramuscularly (i.m.) 0.1 ml/100 gram BW, i.e. 15 mg/kg, 5 times a week for a period of 4 weeks. Control rats received i.m. injections with an identical volume of olive oil vehicle only.

Statistics

Differences in the mean values between the CyA treated rats and controls were compared by Student t-tests. A $p < 0.05$ was considered to be significantly different. To compare effects of CyA between the various models, the GFR of CyA-treated rats was expressed as a percentage of the controls within the same model. Differences between the means of these values in either adult or young rats were compared by oneway analysis of variance and the Newman-Keuls test.

RESULTS

Adult rats

Table I gives the longitudinal changes in BW and GFR occurring during 4 weeks of CyA or vehicle administration in adult rats in relation to the surgical interventions. In adult rats with two intact kidneys (2K), the GFR of CyA treated rats was only slightly less than that of control 2K rats. After one week of treatment the GFR was 13% less, while after 4 weeks of treatment this difference amounted to 24%. Three weeks after cessation of the CyA administration the GFR was similar to that of 2K control rats.

The effects of CyA administration were more outspoken in NX rats than in the 2K rats. The control NX rats showed the compensatory increase in GFR from 50% to 70% of the 2K control level by the 4th postoperative week. The CyA treated NX rats, however, did not have this compensatory increase. The GFR remained at a level of about 50% of that of the 2K rats. Consequently, the differences between CyA and control NX rats increased with time. After the first week the GFR was 21% less, while after 4 weeks the difference had increased to 41%. After cessation of the CyA administration the NX rats showed a rapid increase in the GFR. Six weeks later the GFR was similar to that of control NX rats.

The most pronounced effects of CyA were found in IS+NX rats. Control IS+NX rats showed the expected recovery of the GFR from the ischemic damage as well as the compensatory increase in the GFR of a single remaining kidney. In sharp contrast, the CyA treated IS+NX rats showed almost no increase in their GFR during the treatment course. As a consequence the difference in the GFR from that of control IS+NX rats increased with time. After one week the GFR was 47% less, after 4 weeks this figure amounted to 61%. The GFR did recover after the cessation of the CyA administration, but this recovery was only partial. The greatest increase in the GFR was noted during the first week after cessation of CyA administration. At the end of the follow-up period the GFR was still 30% less than that of control IS+NX rats.

In order to compare the differences in the effects of CyA on the GFR between the various models and to reduce the effects of changes in weight gain, we analyzed

TABLE I

Longitudinal changes in BW and GFR of adult rats treated with ciclosporin.

GROUPS OF RATS	(n)	PRE-TREATMENT BW (gram)	WEEK 1 BW (gram)	WEEK 1 GFR (ml/min)	WEEK 2 BW (gram)	WEEK 2 GFR (ml/min)	WEEK 4 BW (gram)	WEEK 4 GFR (ml/min)
2K–Veh	(6)	270±19	289±22	2.31±0.19	300±24	2.56±0.21	340±40	2.90±0.39
2K–CyA	(7)	269±13	277±18	2.00±0.24#	281±16	2.06±0.24#	309±22	2.20±0.16
NX–Veh	(7)	295±38	298±32	1.57±0.10	311±29	1.67±0.07	346±26	1.94±0.12
NX–CyA	(8)	290±39	279±31	1.24±0.18#	296±24	1.17±0.19#	3.16±24#	1.14±0.23#
IS+NX–Veh	(7)	299±33	277±36	0.87±0.30	301±29	1.15±0.39	331±36	1.54±0.36
IS+NX–CyA	(6)	282±40	239±35#	0.46±0.14#	260±24#	0.48±0.14#	282±30#	0.60±0.09#

GROUPS OF RATS	WEEK 5 BW (gram)	WEEK 5 GFR (ml/min)	WEEK 7 BW (gram)	WEEK 7 GFR (ml/min)	WEEK 10 BW (gram)	WEEK 10 GFR (ml/min)
2K–Veh	ND		387±36	2.82±0.13	ND	
2K–CyA	ND		358±23	2.67±0.33	ND	
NX–Veh	369±27	2.10±0.25	408±27	2.25±0.14	440±26	2.29±0.33
NX–CyA	345±28	1.59±0.19#	385±25	1.95±0.16#	412±17#	2.20±0.23
IS+NX–Veh	362±36	1.64±0.37	406±38	2.06±0.14	426±39	2.23±0.26
IS+NX–CyA	313±34#	1.03±0.10#	365±29	1.36±0.11#	405±19	1.56±0.06

All data are MEAN ± S.D. # $P<0.05$ from vehicle-treated.
ND = not determined; 2K = sham operated two-kidney rats; NX = unilaterally nephrectomized rats; IS+NX = rats that underwent 45 min of renal ischemia and contralateral nephrectomy.

the changes in the GFR (ml/min/100 gram BW) of the CyA treated rats expressed as a percentage of the vehicle-treated animals that had the same surgical intervention. The results of this analysis are depicted in Figure 1A. It is obvious that the nephrotoxicity of CyA was least in the 2K rats and most marked in the IS+NX rats, with an intermediate effect in the NX rats.

Young rats

Table II gives the results in the young rats. In young 2K rats the GFR of CyA-treated animals was about 25% below that of controls after one week of CyA adminitration. No further reduction was noted after 4 weeks of CyA treatment. Apart from a reduction in the developmental increase in the GFR, CyA-treated 2K rats had an impaired growth. At the end of the treatment course, the BW of CyA-treated rats was only 85% of that of controls. This difference in BW remained after cessation of the CyA administration. The difference in GFR became less after cessation of CyA and was comparable to the difference in BW.

In NX rats, CyA had only little effect on the development of the compensatory functional response after unilateral nephrectomy. At the end of the 4 week treatment period the GFR amounted to 83% of that of control NX rats. As with the 2K

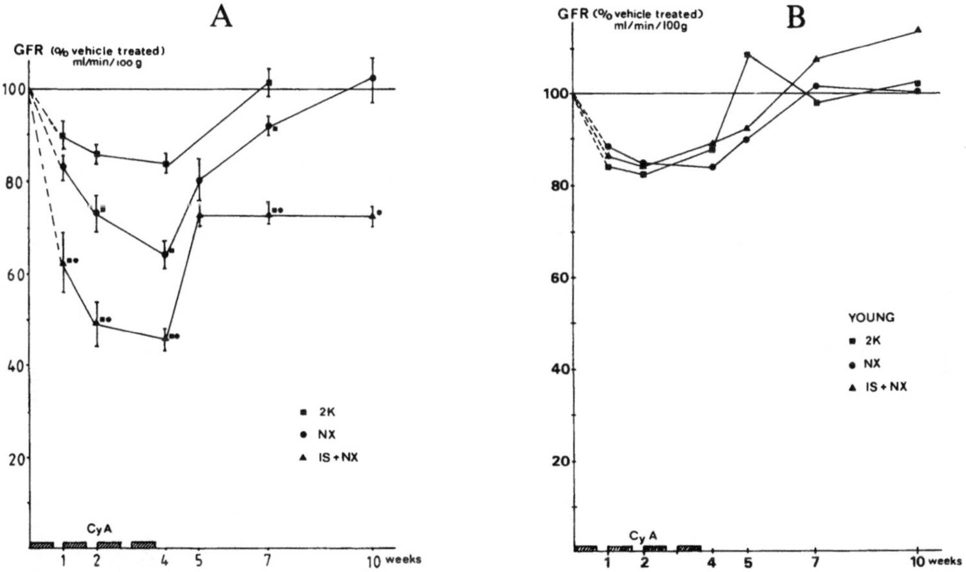

Fig. 1. Longitudinal changes in the GFR of adult (1A) and weanling (1B) rats treated with ciclosporin for 4 weeks. The data represent the mean ± SEM of the GFR (ml/min/100 g BW) expressed as a percentage of the vehicle treated rats that had the same surgical intervention. Symbols are: Squares, sham-operated two-kidney (2K) rats; Circles, unilaterally nephrectomized (NX) rats; Triangles, rats with a single kidney damaged by temporary renal ischemia (IS+NX).

The small symbols indicate significant ($p < 0.05$) differences from rats identified with that symbol.

TABLE II

Longitudinal changes in BW and GFR of weanling rats treated with ciclosporin.

GROUPS OF RATS	(n)	PRE-TREATMENT BW (gram)	WEEK 1 BW (gram)	WEEK 1 GFR (ml/min)	WEEK 2 BW (gram)	WEEK 2 GFR (ml/min)	WEEK 4 BW (gram)	WEEK 4 GFR (ml/min)
2K–Veh	(8)	42±4	67±7	0.66±0.14	101± 8	1.15±0.20	177±15	1.75±0.31
2K–CyA	(8)	43±5	62±9	0.50±0.12#	92±11	0.85±0.15#	151±14	1.30±0.26#
NX–Veh	(8)	45±4	67±5	0.47±0.04	100± 8	0.79±0.08	165±20	1.35±0.18
NX–CyA	(6)	47±3	66±3	0.41±0.06#	94± 6	0.67±0.20	151±17	1.03±0.27#
IS+NX–Veh	(6)	47±4	67±3	0.54±0.04	105± 5	0.86±0.12	174±11	1.35±0.13
IS+NX–CyA	(6)	44±4	56±4	0.39±0.04#	78± 8#	0.53±0.08#	126±14#	0.87±0.12#

GROUP OF RATS	WEEK 5 BW (gram)	WEEK 5 GFR (ml/min)	WEEK 7 BW (gram)	WEEK 7 GFR (ml/min)	WEEK 10 BW (gram)	WEEK 10 GFR (ml/min)
2K–Veh	211±7	1.89±0.24	301±23	2.54±0.21	331±26	2.55±0.25
2K–CyA	191±19	1.84±0.22	275±27	2.26±0.26#	305±9	2.40±0.08
NX–Veh	204±26	1.59±0.18	268±37	1.84±0.22	332±39	2.05±0.16
NX–CyA	187±30	1.32±0.29	250±43	1.75±0.47	315±45	1.99±0.37
IS+NX–Veh	213±17	1.53±0.13	274±21	2.00±0.19	330±27	1.96±0.13
IS+NX–CyA	153±26#	1.03±0.38#	217±19#	1.70±0.14#	276±26#	1.86±0.18

All data are MEAN ± S.D. # $P<0.05$ from vehicle-treated.
2K = sham operated two-kidney rats; NX = unilaterally nephrectomized rats; IS+NX = rats that underwent 45 min of renal ischemia and contralateral nephrectomy.

rats, growth was impaired during CyA treatment. After cessation of treatment, the GFR of CyA treated rats increased to the same level as that of controls.

In IS+NX rats, CyA caused a marked impairment of both body growth and development of the GFR. After one week of treatment, BW was 16% below that of controls and the GFR fell short by 28%. After four weeks BW was 28% and GFR 36% below control levels. Three weeks after cessation of the CyA administration both BW and GFR of the CyA treated animals were about 15–20% less than that of vehicle-treated IS+NX rats.

After excluding the influence of divergent body growth a comparison of the differences in the effect of CyA on the GFR between the various models, showed only little influence of the various operations. During the CyA treatment of 2K rats, NX rats as well as IS+NX rats the GFR (ml/min/100 g BW) was about 75–80% of that of control animals that had undergone the same surgical procedure. From three weeks after cessation of treatment, the GFR relative to BW of CyA-treated rats was no longer different from that of controls (see Figure 1B).

DISCUSSION

The results of the present experiments indicate that there is little difference between the nephrotoxic effects of CyA in adult and young rats with two intact kidneys. In both adult and young rats, the GFR per 100 gram BW of CyA treated animals was about 15% less than that of vehicle treated ones. This indicates that the intrinsic nephrotoxicity of CyA is about the same in young and adult kidneys. Furthermore, the results show that the normal development of renal function during growth is not severely affected by CyA. The normal increase of the GFR was reduced, but this only slightly outranged the reduction in body growth induced by CyA. Such a finding of an equal nephrotoxic effect of CyA in young and adult rats with two intact kidneys contrasts with results observed with other nephrotoxic drugs. We have previously found that equal doses of either aminoglycosides (gentamicin and amikicin) or cis-platin were less nephrotoxic in young than in adult rats [6,7]. This may point to a difference in the nephrotoxic mechanism between the various drugs. For aminoglycosides and cis-platin proximal tubular damage seems important [6,8,9], while vasoconstriction of the afferent arterioles could play a role in the nephrotoxicity of CyA [10].

There are clear differences, however, between the nephrotoxic effects of CyA in adult and young rats with single, compromised kidneys. In adult rats treated with CyA, the percentage of reduction in the GFR as compared with controls was much larger with either intact or ischemically damaged single kidneys remaining after unilateral nephrectomy than with paired intact kidneys. This was not the case in young rats. In adult rats, CyA appears to interfere with the compensatory response after unilateral nephrectomy as well as with the process of recovery normally occurring after an ischemic insult. In contrast, in young animals such an interference does not seem to occur. This may point to a difference in the response to ischemia and/or unilateral nephrectomy between young and adult rats. There is indeed a difference in the rate of recovery from renal ischemia between the young and adult rats. In this experiment, as well as in previous ones (Wessel and Provoost, unpublished data) we have shown that young rats do recover more rapidly than adult rats. One week after applying 45 min of warm ischemia, the GFR of adult kidneys had recovered to about 55% of that of intact kidneys. Young kidneys, however, had completely recovered after one week. Age-dependent differences in the compensatory response of the remaining kidney after unilateral nephrectomy have als been established [11,12,13]. The rat is born after 21 days of gestation with a rather immature kidney. Nephrogenesis continues until at least one week after birth [13], and nephrons develop in a centrifugal way from the juxtamedullary region to the superficial renal cortex. From determinations of the RNA, DNA, and protein content, the renal growth cycle has been divided into three phases [14]. The first phase extends from birth to day 14 and is characterized by hyperplasia. During the second phase, up till day 40, renal growth occurs by a combination of hyperplasia and hypertrophy. In the third phase, after day 40, the kidney grows mainly by hypertrophy. The compensatory response of the remaining kidney after unilateral nephrectomy varies with the age of the animal. Based on measurements of the changes in the RNA/DNA ratio in the renal cortex, it was concluded that hyperplasia plays a more prominent role in the increase in renal mass of young than in adult rats [11]. In adult rats, 80% of the compensatory renal enlargement after UNX can be ascribed to cellular hypertrophy [15].

In contrast to adult kidneys, cells from immature kidneys are already involved in a process of hypertrophy or hyperplasia and as such, the initiation of a compensatory response in immature kidneys might differ from that in adult ones. If such a difference exists, this may explain the difference in the effect of CyA on this response between young and adult kidneys. From the effect in young 2K-rats it is clear that CyA has little effect on normal renal growth. In these growing kidneys, extra compensatory growth induced by contralateral nephrectomy is not affected. Consequently, after the removal of an immature kidney, CyA does not interfere with the initiation of the compensatory growth response.

Provided these experimental findings in rats can be extrapolated to the human situation, the difference in the nephrotoxic response between young and adult kidneys may have consequences in clinical renal transplantation. In that case, less nephrotoxicity is to be expected from CyA in pediatric renal transplantation. If an adult kidney is transplanted into a child, little or no compensatory response is necessary for the functional adaptation to the body size of the recipient [16,17]. On the other hand when an immature kidney is transplanted CyA would not interfere with the compensatory response. Consequently, a normal functional response is to be expected.

In conclusion, the nephrotoxic effect of CyA is about the same in young and adult rats with two intact kidneys. In contrast, after unilateral nephrectomy or ischemic renal damage the immature, growing kidney appears less vulnerable to the nephrotoxic side effects of CyA than an adult kidney.

ACKNOWLEDGEMENT

The author would like to thank Mr. Matthijs van Aken for his technical assistance and Mrs. Alice Ribbink-Goslinga for her editorial assistance.

REFERENCES

1 Calne R.Y., White D.J.G., Thiru S., Evans D.B., McMaster P., Dunn D.C., Craddock G.N., Pentlow B.D., Rolles K. Cyclosporin A in patients receiving renal allografts from cadaver donors. Lancet 1978; ii:1323–1327.
2 Starzl T.E., Weil R., Iwatsuki S., Klintmalm G., Schroeter G.P.J., Koep L.J., Iwaki Y., Terasaki P.I., Porter K.A. The use of cyclosporin A and prednisolone in cadaver kidney transplantation. Surg. Gynecol. Obstet. 1980; 151:17–26.
3 Ryffel B. Experimental toxicological studies with Cyclosporin A. In: Cyclosporin A. D.J.G. White (Ed), Elsevier Biomedical, Amsterdam, 1982; pp. 45–75.
4 Blair J.T., Thomson A.W., Whiting P.H., Davidson R.J.L., Simpson J.G. Toxicity of the immune suppressant Cyclosporin A in the rat. J. Pathol. 1982; 138:163–178.
5 Provoost A.P., De Keijzer M.H., Wolff E.D., Molenaar J.C. Development of renal function in the rat. The measurement of GFR and ERPF and correlation to body and kidney weight. Renal Physiol. 1983; 6:1–9.
6 Provoost A.P., Adejuyigbe O., Wolff E.D. Nephrotoxicity of aminoglycosides in young and adult rats. Ped. Res. 1985; 19:1191–1196.
7 Jongejan H.T.M., Provoost A.P., Wolff E.D., Molenaar J.C. Nephrotoxicity of Cisplatin comparing young and adult rats. Ped. Res. 1986; 20:9–14.
8 Kosek J.D., Mazze R.I., Cousins M.J. Nephrotoxicity of gentamicin. Lab. Invest. 1974; 30:48–57.
9 Chopra S., Kaufman J.S., Jones T.W., Hong W.K., Gehr M.K., Hamburger R.J., Flamenbaum W., Trump B.F. Cis-diamminedichloroplatinum-induced acute renal failure in the rat. Kidney Int. 1982; 21:54–64.
10 Murray B.M., Paller M.S., Ferris T.F. Effect of cyclosporine administration on renal hemodynamics in conscious rats. Kidney Int. 1985; 28:767–774.
11 Dicker S.E., Shirley D.G. Compensatory renal growth after unilateral nephrectomy in the new-born rat. J. Physiol. (Lond.) 1973; 228:193–202.
12 Kaufman J.M., Hardy R., Hayslett J.P. Age-dependent characteristics of compensatory renal growth. Kidney Int. 1975; 8:21–26.
13 Larsson L., Aperia A., Wilton P. Effect of normal development on compensatory renal growth. Kidney Int. 1980; 18:29–35.
14 Winnick M., Noble A. Quantitative changes in DNA, RNA, and protein during prenatal and postnatal growth in the rat. Dev. Biol. 1966; 12:451–466.
15 Johnson H.A., Vera Roman J.M. Compensatory renal enlargement: Hypertrophy vs. hyperplasia. Amer. J. Pathol. 1966; 49:1–13.
16 Provoost A.P., De Keijzer M.H., Kort W.J., Van Aken M., Weijma I.M., Wolff E.D., Molenaar

J.G. The influence of the recipient upon renal function after isogeneic kidney transplantation in the rat. Transplantation 1984; 37:55–62.

17 Provoost A.P., Wolff E.D., De Keijzer M.H., Molenaar J.C. Influence of the recipients's size upon renal function following kidney transplantation. An experimental and clinical investigation. J. Pediatr. Surg. 1984; 19:63–67.

TWO YEARS EXPERIENCE IN THE USE OF CICLOSPORIN IN RENAL TRANSPLANTATION IN CHILDREN

T.K. MATTOO, S.P.A. RIGDEN, G.B. HAYCOCK, C. CHANTLER, A. MUNIAN, C.G. KOFFMAN and M. BEWICK

Evelina Children's Hospital, Guy's Hospital, London, England.

In our experience the use of CyA is associated with a lower incidence of graft loss due to rejection and a marked reduction in the incidence and severity of corticosteroid related side effects. However, the overall graft survival was not improved mainly because of the high incidence of vascular complications occurring in kidneys from donors aged less than 6 years. CyA therapy is associated with a reversible reduction in GFR in the majority of patients, but we do not recommend conversion from CyA to AZA because of the significant risk of rejection occurring on withdrawal of CyA.

Ciclosporin (CyA), in combination with low dose steroid therapy and in some patients azathioprine (AZA), has been given to all children receiving renal transplants at Guy's Hospital since October 1983.

MATERIALS AND METHODS

In the two year period 01/10/83 to 30/09/85 forty-one boys and 25 girls aged from 9 months to 17 years received 79 renal allografts (Fig.1): the results were analysed on 01/04/86. Eight boys and 4 girls were retransplanted during the study period. Seven patients were less than 5 years old, one of whom received 3 grafts. There were 4 live related donor grafts (all first transplants, 3 from parents and 1 from a paternal uncle) and 75 cadaver grafts, of which 46 were first grafts, 23 second and 6 third grafts. The mean age of the cadaver graft donors was 10.6 years, range 1-48 years with 53% being less than 6 years old. Negative cross match and identical blood groups were the only criteria for accepting first grafts.

CyA regimes

The 3 CyA regimes used during this period are summarised in Table I. CyA was given by mouth with the first dose being given 1 hour preoperatively. Trough levels of CyA were measured in whole blood using radioimmunoassay. All patients were given

Correspondence to: S.P.A. Rigden, Evelina Children's Hospital, 9th floor Guy's Tower, Guy's Hospital, London. SE1 9RT, England

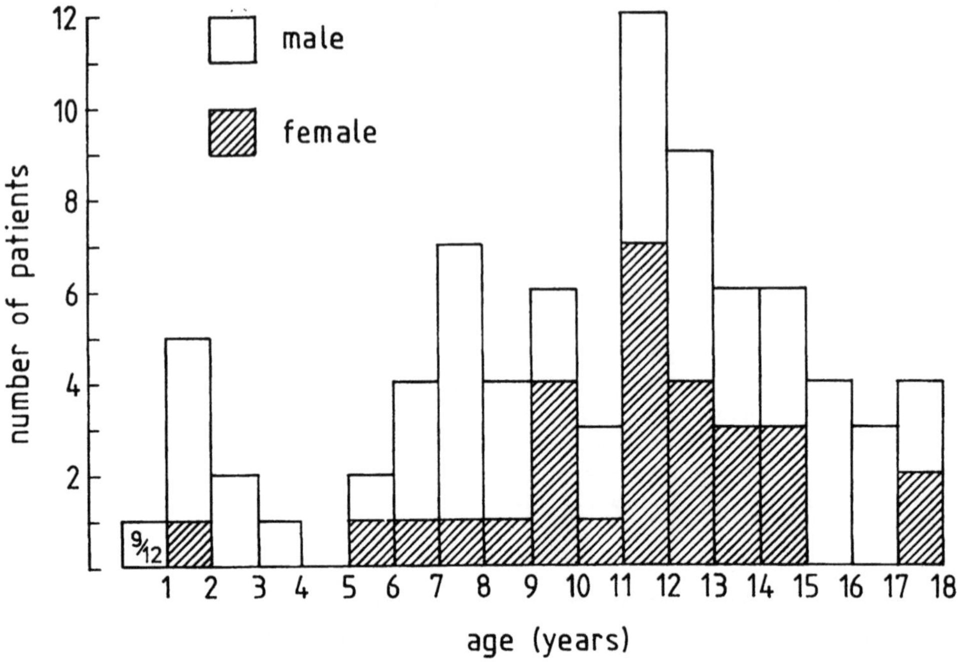

Fig.1. Age of the 66 recipients at the time of the transplant (79 grafts).

TABLE I

CyA Regimes

	07/10/83-30/06/84	01/07/84-30/09/84	01/10/84-30/09/85
1 hour pre-operatively	150 mg/m^2	300 mg/m^2	> 2 yrs 450 mg/m^2 < 2 yrs 600 mg/m^2
12 hours post-operatively	150 mg/m^2	300 mg/m^2	> 2 yrs 450 mg/m^2 < 2 yrs 600 mg/m^2
followed by	150 mg/m^2 x 2/day	150 mg/m^2 x 2/day	300 mg/m^2 x 2/day x 5 days 200 mg/m^2 x 2/day x 5 days 150 mg/m^2 x 2/day
aiming for trough CyA levels of	400 μg/l month 1 200-400 μg/l thereafter	400--800 μg/l month 1 200-400 μg/l thereafter	600–800 μg/l week 1 400-600 μg/l week 2 200-400 μg/l thereafter

methylprednisolone (MeP) 600 mg/m^2 body surface area intravenously one hour pre-operatively, followed by oral prednisolone 5 mg/m^2 twice daily for one month, after which the dose was reduced to 5 mg/m^2 once daily for a further month and finally to 10 mg/m^2 on alternate days indefinitely. Patients receiving second or third transplants and those with cytotoxic antibodies were given Fresenius antithymocyte globulin (ATG) 2 mg/kg intravenously pre-operatively and daily for 9 days post-operatively. During the third CyA regime AZA 60 mg/m^2 was also given starting on the first post-operative day or on the seventh post-operative day in those children receiving ATG. The rationale being that the addition of AZA might reduce the requirement for CyA, thereby reducing nephrotoxicity.

Acute rejection episodes occurring during the first six weeks post transplant were treated with intravenous MeP 600 mg/m^2 on three consecutive days: after six weeks oral prednisolone was given in a dose of 3 mg/kg/day for three consecutive days. If the response was incomplete after the three days treatment, a further 3 doses of intravenous MeP or oral prednisolone were given on alternate days.

Complications

CyA therapy was discontinued in 30 children: in 2 abruptly because of severe nephrotoxicity, while in the other 28 it was gradually withdrawn, six to twelve months post-transplant over 8-10 weeks, after increasing the dose of prednisolone to 30 mg/m^2 on alternate days and starting AZA 60 mg/m^2 daily in those children not already taking it. This protocol was abandoned on 31/12/85.

One patient, a boy aged 7 years, died of Serratia septicemia three weeks after his first graft which had primary non-function and biopsy proven acute rejection. Two further children died some months after being returned to hemodialysis following graft loss.

Graft survival

One of the live related grafts has been lost at 81 weeks due to chronic rejection. Actuarial survival of 1st and 2nd cadaveric grafts is shown in Figure 2. Three of the six third cadaver grafts have been lost: one to chronic rejection at 33 weeks, and the other two were found to be infarcted early in the post operative course. The other three are functioning at 130, 39 and 30 weeks respectively. The one year actuarial survival of first cadaver grafts of 67% is rather disappointing when compared with 76% one year survival for all cadaver grafts performed in the same unit during the period 1981–1983 using steroids and AZA immunosuppression. Possible reasons for this emerge from examining the causes of graft loss (Table II). The incidence of loss due to acute rejection was very low (2/26). Seven grafts were lost because of chronic rejection, though one of these children was known to have been non-compliant with his drugs and in another immunosuppression was discontinued for a period of time because of chickenpox. Three further children lost their grafts in association with severe infections.

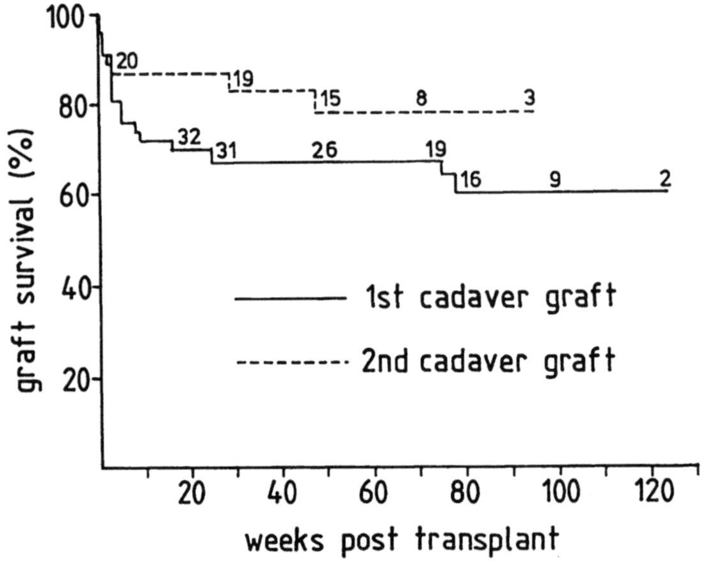

Fig.2. Actuarial survival for first (46) and second (23) cadaver grafts 01/10/83 to 30/09/85 analysed 01/04/86. The numbers of patients at risk are shown along the lines.

TABLE II

Causes of graft loss	total 26
Acute rejection	2
Chronic rejection	7**
Infections/rejection	
CMV/UTI	1
severe viral illness*	1
Serratia septicemia* +	1
Vascular accidents	
venous thrombosis and infarction	4
transplant artery occlusion acute	2
transplant artery anastomosis rupture	2
failure to establish perfusion at operation: nephrectomy	1
Lost during surgical repair of	
transplant artery stenosis	2
lower ureteric obstruction	1
Hemorrhage post-biopsy	1
Acute CyA toxicity	1

* immunosuppression withdrawn

** includes one patient in whom immunosuppression was withdrawn for a period, one non-compliant patient and one live related donor graft

\+ patient died

Vascular problems

Eleven grafts were lost due to vascular problems: 10 of them came from donors aged less than 6 years (10/40 v 1/35: $\chi^2 = 7.3$. $p < 0.01$). Losses due to all other causes were not more common in kidneys from donors aged less than 6 years (8/40 v 6/35: $\chi^2 = 0.1$. NS). In addition to the two kidneys lost during attempted surgical repair of transplant artery stenosis, ten further children have been found on renal arteriography to have transplant artery stenosis. Two children have undergone successful surgical repair, 2 have been improved by percutaneous angioplasty and the remaining 6 have had their blood pressure controlled medically without deterioration in renal function in 5. Initially there was concern that this high incidence of transplant artery stenosis was a complication of CyA therapy, but 10 out of the 12 affected kidneys were harvested from donors aged less than 6 years whereas only 2 stenoses occurred in the 35 kidneys from older donors (10/40 v 2/35: $\chi^2 = 5.17$ $p < 0.05$). Retrospective analysis of the last 65 grafts performed in our unit using prednisolone and AZA as immunosuppression, prior to the introduction of CyA revealed the same problem. There were 7 cases of renal artery stenosis. 5 of which occurred in donors aged less than 6 years. Of the 65 donors only 12 were aged less than 6 years (5/12 v 2/53: $\chi^2 = 14.6$. $p < 0.001$). Thus renal artery stenosis appears to be a hazard of the use of kidneys from donors aged less than 6 years, independent of the immunosuppressive agents used.

Nephrotoxicity

In 30 children CyA was withdrawn because of concerns about long term nephrotoxicity. Eight (27%) children developed acute rejection episodes either during the withdrawal period or shortly after CyA had been discontinued and all required reinstitution at therapeutic levels. No kidneys were lost because of this, though most had some irreversible loss of renal function. Of those in whom CyA was discontinued successfully, 21 had chromium EDTA GFR determinations before and after its withdrawal. There was a mean rise in GFR of 10 ml/min/1.73 m^2 SA suggesting that CyA does cause a depression in GFR. In one child CyA was discontinued abruptly because of rapidly deteriorating renal function and renal biopsy appearances suggestive of acute CyA nephrotoxicity despite low CyA whole blood levels. His renal function began to improve and now 13 months later he has a plasma creatinine of 55 μmol/l.

FIVE YEARS EXPERIENCE WITH CICLOSPORIN TREATMENT AFTER RENAL TRANSPLANTATION IN CHILDREN

B. KLARE, H. HAHN, E. MEUSEL, M. STEINHOFF, P. EMMRICH[1], W. LAND[2]

[1]*Children's Clinic and Polyclinic, Technical University of Munich, 8000 München 40, Federal Republic of Germany*
[2]*Transplantation Centre, Surgical Clinic, Klinikum Großhadern, University of Munich*

For the last 5 years we have made 19 renal transplantations with subsequent CyA therapy in 16 children aged 4 months to 17 years. 8 patients were followed for more than two years, 6 for more than 3 years. In order to obtain better growth we decided to use CyA instead of the conventional therapy with AZA and daily steroids. At the beginning of therapy, 15–30 mg CyA/kg BW were needed to achieve blood levels of 300–400 ng/ml. In general, higher dosage/kg BW was required in smaller children. Steroids were withdrawn after 6 months. Since July 84 we additionally gave AZA 2 mg/kg initially for 1–2 weeks. Patient survival was 100%. Before drug monitoring was possible we had 70% 5-year graft survival, while after monitoring of CyA levels 3-year graft survival was 90%. Rejection episodes occurred rarely compared to AZA/steroids, only when the CyA level fell below 200 ng/ml. The most helpful parameters to distinguish between rejection episodes and nephrotoxicity were the increase of CyA level and of serum uric acid in nephrotoxicity, but normalising of serum uric acid in rejection episodes. All children (except one) had at least normal, or even catch-up growth. Two other children with reduced growth after renal transplantation were converted from AZA/steroids to CyA and started growing again.

With the introduction of ciclosporin (CyA) in 1978 in Europe and in 1980 in the USA, results of renal transplantation obtained in adults improved decisively. Compared with the conventional therapy with azathioprine (AZA) and steroids, the 1-year transplant survival rate rose by over 15% and the patient survival rate by more than 5% [1,2].

Rejection episodes were less frequently observed than in conventional therapy. The idea of using CyA also in paediatric patients, was especially attractive, because steroids could than be avoided. Most difficulties of transplanted children result from steroid side effects. The need for steroids in particular continues the problem of growth retardation, which is the most severe long term problem for children with chronic renal failure [3,4,5]. In 1981 we decided very early in the context of the European multicentre study [1] to introduce CyA for children because we

Correspondence to: B. Klare, Children's Clinic and Polyclinic, Technical University of Munich, 8000 München 40, Federal Republic of Germany hoped that normal body growth would occur with the possibility of complete social rehabilitation.

MATERIAL

Since March 1981 we did 19 cadaver renal transplantations with CyA in 16 children. The age ranged from 0.3 to 17 years. The therapy regimen of CyA was modified four times (Table I). From March 1981 to June 1982, 8 children were given 15 mg/kg body weight (BW) CyA, tapering to 6 mg/kg within 6 months. Since March 1983 when the monitoring of CyA blood levels was introduced, we increased CyA dosage to 25–30 mg/kg BW [3]. Later on we administered 500 mg CyA/m^2 body-surface area initially [6]. Afterwards the dosage was corrected, sometimes daily, to maintain the appropriate blood level of 500 ng/ml. In July 1984 AZA 2 mg/kg BW was given additionally for 1–2 weeks until CyA levels were stable. Since January 1985 we have lowered the desired CyA trough level to 250 ng/ml to reduce nephrotoxicity.

The first 3 children never had steroids. Five received only 8 mg/1.73 m^2 prednisone initially, which we reduced rapidly within 4 weeks. After 6 months steroids were discontinued.

In 1982 we converted 2 children from AZA/steroids to CyA, because of growth retardation for more than one year. In both the prednisone dose was 5 mg/day. At 8 months after conversion, steroids were discontinued.

In episodes of suspected rejection, boluses of 10 mg/kg BW methylprednisolone were given for 3 days. In difficult situations it was given for 6 days, with a reduction to 5 mg/kg from the 4th to the 6th day. In all cases CyA dosage was increased after taking a blood sample to be used to measure the CyA target level. If 2 rejection therapies with only methylprednisolone were unsuccessful we used to give anti-lymphocyte globulin. This was replaced by antithymocyte globulin in the last year, which was given combined with 5 mg/kg BW methylprednisolone for 7 days.

RESULTS

Patient survival was 100%. The mean follow-up for 19 renal transplants was 1.8 years. The 5-year graft survival rate was 70% including the early phase without monitoring of CyA levels. Since the introduction of CyA blood level monitoring, the graft survival rate has increased to 90% after 3 years (Fig. 1). The first blood level measurements, with the maintenance dosage of 6 mg/kg BW, showed CyA levels below 100 ng/ml- in all 6 examined children. This dosage from the protocol of the European multicentre study [1] proved to be too low for children [3,6]. Subsequently we increased the CyA dose to achieve the desired level of 500 ng/ml. Since 1985 we have aimed to obtain levels of only 250 ng/ml, 3 months after transplantation. We found that small children needed a relatively high dose of CyA per kg BW.

TABLE I

Immunosuppressive regimens with Ciclosporin in children after renal transplantation.

changes of treatment regimens	number of renal transplants	CICLOSPORIN dosage, mg initial	6th month	desired trough level ng/ml	AZATHIOPRINE initially for 1–2 weeks	PREDNISONE, mg initial	after 1 month	after 6 month
since March 1981	3	15/kg	6/kg	-	-	0	0	0
since June 1982	5	15/kg	6/kg	-	-	$8/1.73m^2$	$8/1.73m^2$	-
since March 1983	3	25–30/kg	individual*	500	-	$60/m^2$	$9/m^2$	-
Since July 1984	8	$500/m^2$	individual	400**	2 mg/kg	$60/m^2$	$9/m^2$	-

*Dosage individually adjusted to CyA levels
**Since January 1985, 3 months after RT, we adjusted to 250 ng/ml.

Treatment of acute rejection episodes:

1) Boluses of Methylprednisolone 10 mg/kg BW for 3 days, if necessary we continued with 5 mg/kg BW from the 4th to the 6th day.
2) Elevation of the CyA dosage in order to adjust CyA level not lower than 400 ng/ml.

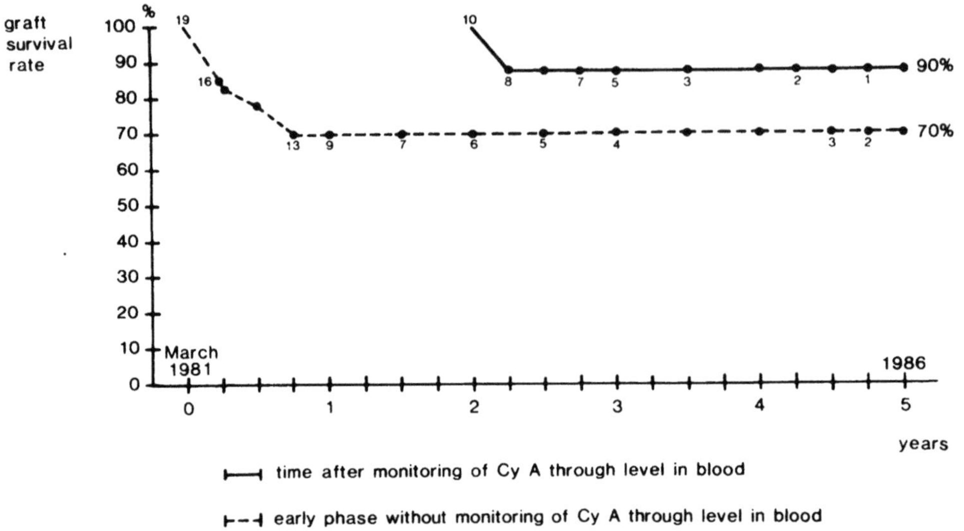

Fig. 1. Graft survival rate with Ciclosporin after 19 renal transplants in 16 children, age 0.3–17 years (March 1986)

Thirty-eight rejection therapies were given to 19 renal transplant recipients corresponding to 1.1/rejection therapies/patient year. The frequency of rejection therapies fell to 0.36/year in 11 patients observed longer than 1 year. After carrying out a retrospective analysis we think that 40% of the rejection therapies were superfluous – because rejection could not be confirmed (Fig. 2). True rejection episodes had occurred in only 11 (58%) of 19 renal transplant recipients, correspond to 1.9/year. One year after renal transplantation 4 of 11 recipients still had 1.1 rejection episode/year. In 7 cases we could not clearly separate one rejection episode from the next one. Therefore we could evaluate only 16 of 23 episodes. The diagnoses were histologically confirmed in 9 cases. The clinical symptoms of these 16 rejection episodes in 11 children were not impressive. There was fever twice. Only 6 of the 16 felt ill or complained of pain in the transplant area (Table II). A transient decrease of the CyA level below 200 ng/ml has been observed in most of the patients.

In 9 out of 12 cases the initially increased serum uric acid level approached normal values, despite a rise in serum creatinine level. With the exception of 4 cases where serum creatinine was more than 4 mg%. In 13 out of 16 episodes an enlargement of graft volume was measured by ultra-sound. Most of these kidneys also showed a pronounced medullary cone, which was not well separated from the renal interstitial tissue. The blood pressure rose during 13 of the 16 rejection episodes.

Retrospectively we found in 15 non confirmed rejection therapies 5 cases of acute tubular necrosis, 4 times an increase of serum creatinine due to CyA toxicity, 4 cases of fluid imbalance after infection or diarrhoea and one interstitial fibrosis

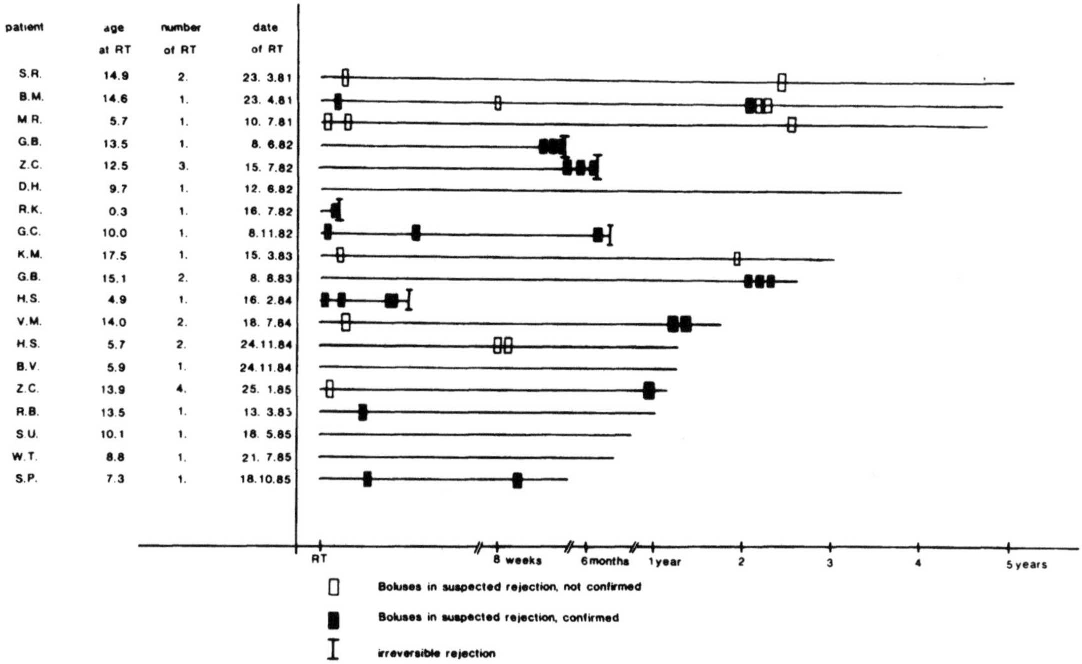

Fig. 2. Moments of rejection therapies (boluses of methylprednisolone) in 19 renal transplantations with Ciclosporin.

of the transplant. Acute tubular necrosis after transplantation occurred more frequently with CyA than in conventional therapy. If the cold ischemic time of donor graft was below 24 hours, 6 of 8 transplants started to function on the first day, while only 4 out of 11 functioned on the first day with a cold ischemic time longer than 24 hours (Table III).

Rejection therapies were sometimes given although the rise of serum creatinine

TABLE II

Symptoms of 16 certain rejection episodes in 11 children with CyA therapy

-	fever	2/16	12%
-	slight illness	6/16	37%
-	slight pain from renal transplant	6/16	37%
-	serum creatinine increased	16/16	100%
-	CyA trough level transitorily <200 ng/ml	12/13	92%
-	uric acid level transitorily decreased	9/12	75%
	(except that serum creatinine >4.0 mg%	4	--
-	enlargement of graft volume sonografically	13/16	81%
-	increase of blood pressure	13/16	81%

TABLE III

Cold ischemic time and start of graft function

Patient	age (years)	ischemic time (h)	start of function
H.S. 1	4.7	16	day 1
S.U.	10.1	20	day 1
S.P.	7.2	20	day 7
H.S. 2	5.8	21	month 4
W.T.	8.8	21	day 1
D.H.	9.8	23	day 1
S.R.	14.9	24	day 1
B.M.	14.6	24	day 1
Z.C. 1	12.4	25	day 17
B.V.	5.9	25	day 1
R.B.	13.5	25	day 13
V.M.	14.0	25	day 49
R.C.	0.3	26	day 1
G.B. 1	13.9	26	day 1
G.B. 2	15.1	28	day 12
Z.C. 2	13.9	34	day 44
K.M.	17.5	35	day 14
G.C.	10.0	40	day 1
M.R.	5.7	41	day 10

was due to nephrotoxicity of CyA. Acute increase of nephrotoxicity did not produce any clinical symptoms. Occasionally we found increased blood pressure and a slight sonographic enlargement of the graft. CyA levels above 400 ng/ml correlated with laboratory signs of renal toxicity. We observed increases of serum creatinine and particulary of serum uric acid above the normal range in most cases. However, 16 out of 19 transplants with CyA levels between 200 and 400 ng/ml also showed increased uric acid levels. Only 3 children had uric acid levels in the normal range, but like all the other children they showed an increase of serum uric acid and serum creatinine with increasing CyA levels (Fig. 3 and 4). On the other hand normal serum uric acid values were measured 5 months after transplantation in the 5 children with CyA underdosage, before monitoring of CyA levels was performed.

One patient transplanted twice, seems to illustrate the diagnostic help of the uric acid level (Fig. 5). The first graft was irreversibly rejected 7 months after RT, before CyA monitoring was available. A few weeks before rejection, slightly elevated serum creatinine and serum uric acid normalised. During rejection, serum creatinine rose whereas uric acid stayed normal. In contrast, with the second graft, we observed a slightly elevated serum creatinine but high serum uric acid levels. This was an

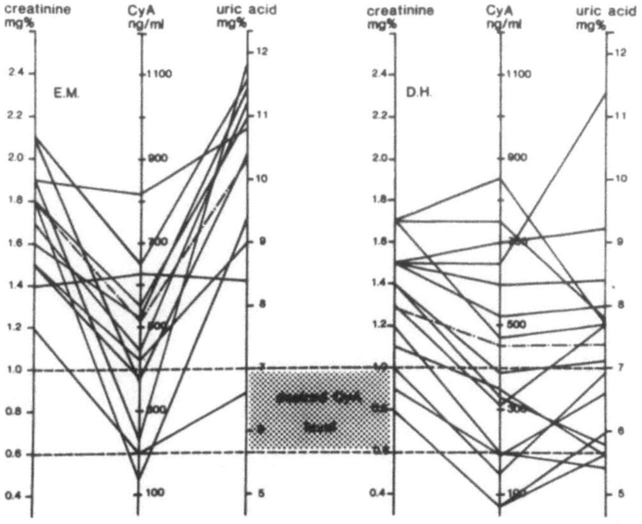

Fig. 3. Serum creatinine and serum uric acid were elevated if CyA trough level was in the desired range between 200 and 400 ng/ml (shaded area). These 2 cases show that increases of creatinine and uric acid are individually different.

argument for nephrotoxicity, although CyA levels had been low, between 50 and 150 ng/ml for 3 months.

Various forms of CyA toxicity have been observed in all children (Table IV). All showed hypertrichosis of varying degrees. In 17 of 18 patients slight to extreme hyperplasia of the gingiva was seen, with apelike prognathism in 2 cases. Ten out of 18 children had a tremor in the first 2 weeks after RT but no other cerebral symptoms. Hypomagnesemia was a prominent feature. All children had signs of nephrotoxicity, i.e. increased serum creatinine and serum uric acid dependant on their CyA level. Both substances decreased after lowering the CyA level from 500 to 250 ng/ml. In spite of this, creatinine and uric acid remained slightly above normal.

Fifteen out of 18 children transiently had serum potassium values above normal in the first month. Most of them also had serum potassium values repeatedly above 5 mMol/l in the following years. One girl had regularly diminished serum potassium levels between 2.8 and 3.3 mMol/L. She had a hemosiderosis and CyA toxicity in spite of a CyA level of only 100 ng/ml.

We found hypomagnesemia in 10 of 11 children investigated in the first weeks after RT, often combined with tremor. Hepatotoxic symptoms were rarely observed.

Hypertension amenable to control by medication was the most frequent acute problem of clinical relevance. In a group of 21 children including two after conversion from AZA to CyA, 4 did not have hypertension. Seventeen (81%) needed 2–5 antihypertensive drugs. All received nifidepine. In 7 cases captopril was given in

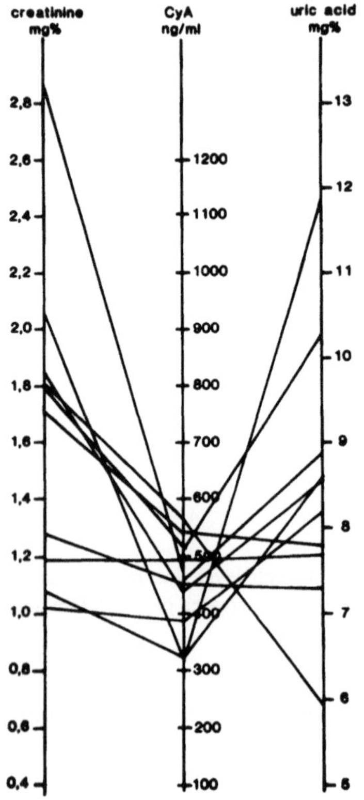

Fig. 4. Mean serum creatinine and mean serum uric acid had individually different increased values in relation to their mean CyA blood level in 10 children.

order to achieve age-related mean normal values of blood pressure. In 7 children who dit not have well controlled hypertension we did angiography because of suspected transplant artery stenosis. This diagnosis was confirmed in 6 cases.

Side effects due to reduced resistance against infections were rare. We observed 11 infections in 7 children, during 34 patient years. One life-threatening urosepsis was noted after rejection therapy with antilymphocyte globulin. All 7 children developing terminal renal insufficiency previously had infectious problems. One child had had bacteremia twice from chapped skin near the Bentley-button of his Bentley-shunt. One child had recurrent diarrhoea due to Lambliasis, one had thrombophlebitis associated with superinfected atopic dermatitis and one had herpes zoster.

Transitorily we saw Cushing's facies in 15 out of 18 children, but no other serious side effects from steroids. We saw no steroid-induced growth retardation. Longitudinal growth resumed, strikingly early. Children who did not receive massive doses of steroids showed catch-up growth (Fig. 6). In some children we saw that catch-up growth apparently stopped with continued normal growth when the individual growth of percentile was reached.

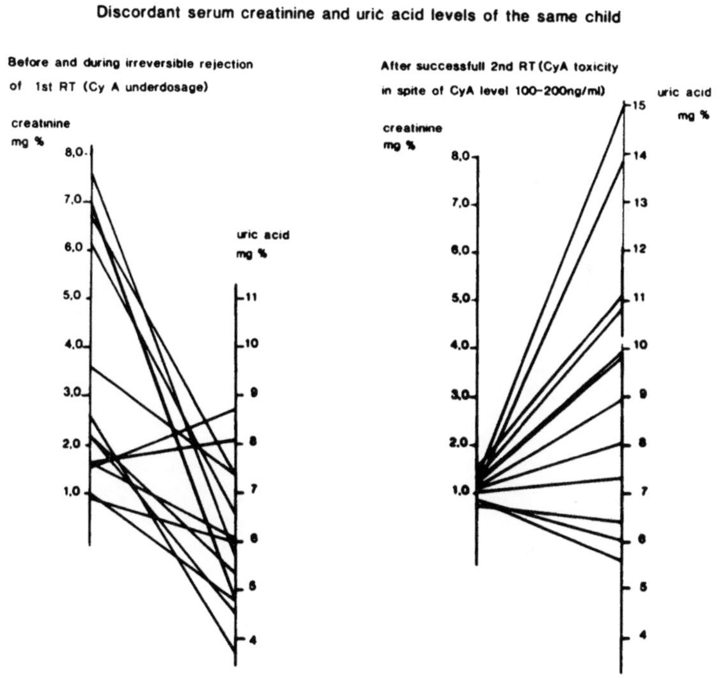

Fig. 5. Reaction of serum creatinine and serum uric acid in one child, twice transplanted with CyA. In the first graft with rejection (left side), serum uric acid dropped to normal when serum creatinine rose. In the second graft serum uric acid increased highly with increasing serum creatinine as a sign of nephrotoxicity.

TABLE IV

Frequency of CyA toxicity symptoms in 18 children.

General symptoms		Nephrotoxic symptoms	
hypertrichosis	18/18	serum creatinine	↑ 17/18
hyperplasia of gingiva	17/18	serum uric acid	↑ 18/18
		serum urea	↑ 18/18
		transitorily serum potassium	↑ 15/18
		transitorily serum magnesium	↓ 9/10
Neurological symptoms		**Hepatotoxic symptoms**	
transitorily tremor	10/18	transitorily bilirubin	↑ 3/18
convulsions	0/18	transitorily cholinesterase	↓ 6/18
other	0		

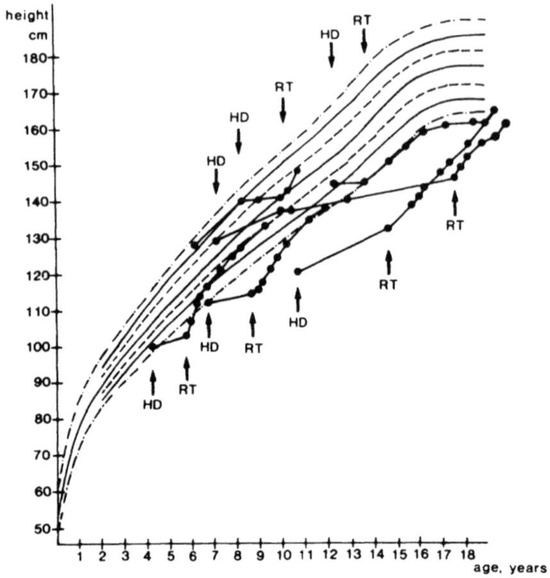

Fig. 6. After renal transplantation with CyA 5 of 6 boys showed catch-up growth up to an age of 19 years. One 13 year old boy had normal growth velocity but not catch-up growth, because chronic renal failure occurred in the transplant. HD = hemodialysis, RT = renal transplantation

Catch-up growth has even been observed in an 18 year old boy with retarded bone age. Normal growth, but not catch-up growth, occurred twice when chronic renal failure recurred, with serum creatinine values above 3 mg%. We observed catch-up growth in two children following conversion to CyA therapy after growth retardation was seen with conventional therapy (Fig. 7).

Only one girl did not grow normally, although steroids were discontinued for more than one year. Until now we have not found the cause. The girl has a haemosiderosis. Eight children (with observation periods of 2 to 5 years) did not show reduction of renal function (Fig.8).

DISCUSSION

Since the introduction of CyA with monitoring of CyA blood levels, graft survival of transplanted children has improved significantly [2,5] compared to results with conventional therapy [7,8]. Only few pediatric centres report a 5-year graft survival of more than 80%, with conventional therapy [9,10]. Our results in 1981 and 1982 without monitoring of CyA were not better than conventionally treated children because underdosage of CyA could not be detected [3].

It seems characteristic that 3 of 4 irreversible rejections occurred 5–7 months after RT, around the time that CyA dosage was reduced to the lowest maintainance

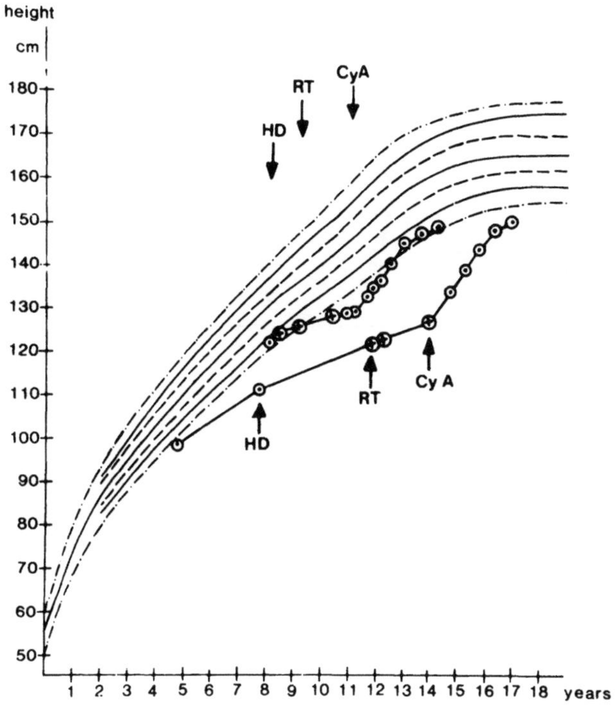

Fig. 7. Body growth of 2 children was retarded during maintainance hemodialysis and after renal transplantations with Azathioprine and steroid (5 mg/d). After conversion to Ciclosporin catch-up growth occurred. HD = hemodialysis, RT = renal transplantation

dose of 6 mg/kg BW. We found that the dosage regimen prescribed for adults was too low for children, because CyA levels were lower than 100 ng/ml in most children. We calculated that smaller children needed higher CyA dosages related to BW, in order to achieve sufficient CyA blood levels. At this point we changed the dosage scheme from one using body weight into one with reference to the body surface area [6]. However, it still was not possible to give a fixed dosage regimen. Because CyA levels fluctuate unpredictably, we recommend daily CyA estimations until a stable level is achieved. We aim during the first 4 weeks for a CyA level of 400 ng/ml (300–500 ng/ml), later on 250 ng/ml (200–300 ng/ml).

Some children have a high risk of rejection, if the CyA level falls below 200 ng/ml. All our comfirmed rejection episodes, except two, and all irreversible rejections reported so far [11, 12, 13], have arisen in the presence of demonstrably reduced CyA levels, or other signs of CyA underdosage. Rejection episodes were less frequent with CyA than with conventional therapy, because some children never

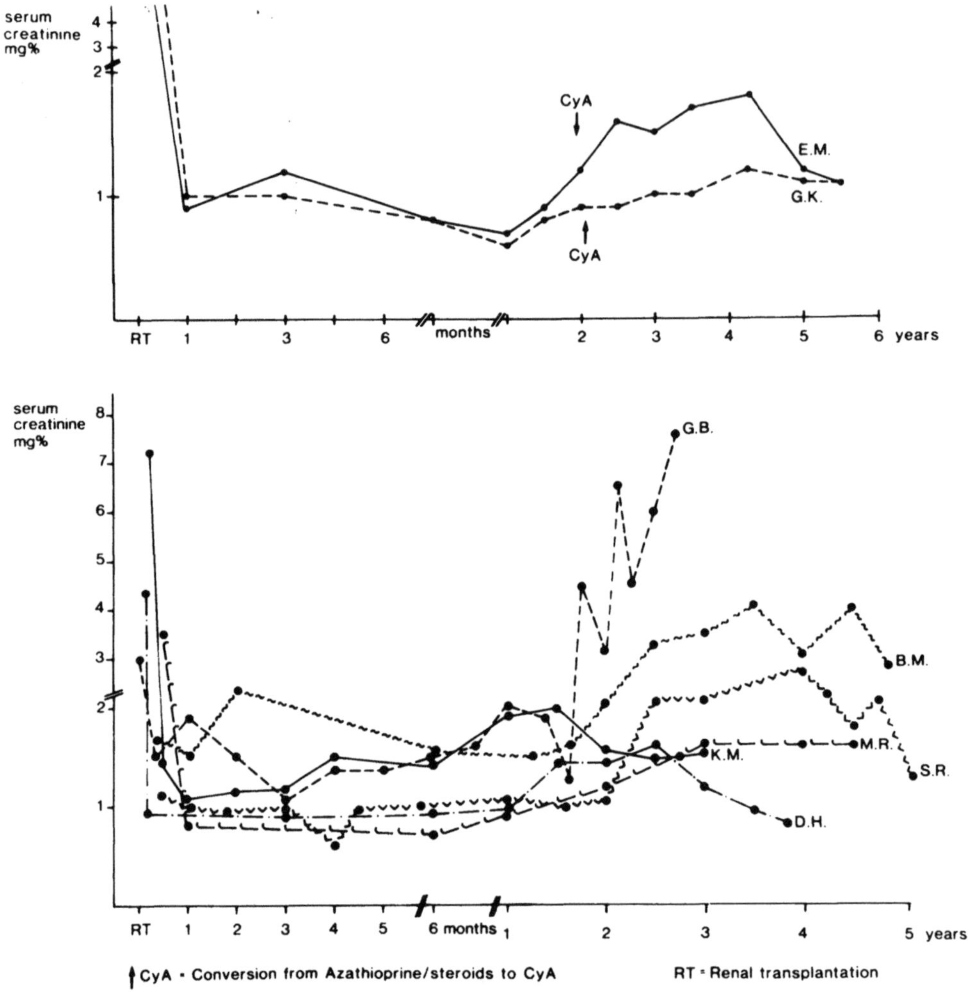

Fig. 8. Follow up after RT with CyA in 8 children observed for more than 2 years. Two of them (top part) were converted from AZA/steroids to CyA two years after transplantation.

About two and a half years ago all 8 children had an increase of serum creatinine, when we increased CyA dose to regulate CyA level on 500 ng/ml. This reduction of renal function was partially reversible in 6 children, when we lowered CyA level to 250 ng/ml about 1.2 years ago. One 16 year old girl (G.B.) unexpectedly had repeated rejection episodes because of repeated non-compliance to CyA treatment. Another child with suspected rejection showed histological rejection and interstitial fibrosis (B.M.). Serum creatinine became stabilized at 3 mg% for more than 2 years.

had a rejection episode. In the first two years after the introduction of CyA our most difficult problem was to distinguish between rejection and nephrotoxicity. The classic clinical symptoms of rejection were often suppressed. Repeatedly we could only make the diagnosis by biopsy. Later on, after introduction of CyA monitoring, we could better recognize CyA toxicity. Furthermore the determination of serum uric acid has been very helpful in the differentiation between rejection and nephrotoxicity.

In the presence of raised serum creatinine attributable to nephrotoxicity, we found the serum uric acid had risen more than corresponded to the reduced glomerular filtration rate. We think that the decreased tubular uric acid secretion is due to the CyA nephrotoxicity. During "rejection", with reduced CyA levels we frequently observed that previously raised uric acid values dropped to normal. This normalization of elevated serum uric acid levels, signals a reduction of CyA toxicity. Wether the immunosuppressive effect of CyA is reduced concomitantly, is not clear. If the CyA levels are above 200 ng/ml, the uric acid levels do not seem to be of critical importance. But the situation is more risky, if CyA levels are too low and the uric acid level is normal or dropping to normal. On the other hand we very cautiously reduced CyA levels to 100 ng/ml in 3 children, when uric acid levels were clearly elevated. One of these children had symptoms of gout as has been reported elsewhere [14]. We emphasize that the tremor associated with hypomagnesemia can be successfully treated with oral magnesium [15].

We discontinued steroids early and think that this practice has contributed to the low rate of infectious complications. Until now we have seen no advantage in using steroids for mai7tainance therapy. We did not see more frequent rejection episodes after discontinuation of steroids. On the contrary, similar to other reports [3, 16, 17], we have experienced the greatest benefit for our children in avoiding steroid induced growth retardation with the chance of catch-up growth in most of them. Demonstrating what we had hoped for, we even observed catch-up growth in 2 boys between 17 and 19 years. Both these young men are now well rehabilitated.

REFERENCES

1 Calne R.Y., Wood A.J., European Multicentre Trial Group. Cyclosporin in cadaveric renal transplantation: 3 year follow-up of a european multicentre trial. Lancet 1985 ii:549.

2 Land W., Castro L.A., White D.J.G., Hillebrand G., Hammer C., Klare B., Fornara P. Cyclosporin in renal transplantation. Progr. in Allergy 1986; 38:293-328.

3 Klare B., von Walter J., Hahn H., Emmrich P., Land W. Cyclosporin in renal transplantation in children. Lancet 1984; ii:692.

4 Fennel R.S.I.I.I., Orak J.K., Hudson T., Garin E.H., Iravani A., Van Deuzen W.J., Howard R., Pfaff W.W., Walker R.D.I.I.I., Richard C.A. Growth in children with various therapies for end-stage renal disease. Am. J. Dis. Childh. 1984; 138:28–31.

5 Offner G. Nierentransplantation im Kindesalter. Dialyse-Journal 1985; 13:50–56.

6 Hoyer P.F., Offner G., Wonigeit K., Brodehl J., Pichelmayr R. Dosage of Cyclosporine A in children with renal transplants. Clin. Nephrol. 1984; 22:68–71.

7 Brodehl J., Pichelmayr R., Offner G. Nierentransplantation bei Kindern. Kinderarzt 1984; 15:1553–1560.

8 Chantler C., Carter J.E., Bewick M., Counahan R., Cameron J.S., Ogg C.S., Williams G., Winder E. 10 years experience with regular hemodialysis and renal transplantation. Arch. Dis. Childh. 1980; 55:435–445.

9 Broyer M., Gagnadoux M.F., Niaudet P. Kidney transplantation in children: results and late sequelae. In: Paediatric Nephrology. Brodehl J., Erich J.H.H. (eds), Springer Verlag, 1984; pp. 138–145.

10 Schärer K., Dreikorn K., Mehls O., Müller-Wiefel D., Ibrsch R., Brittinger W. Spätprognose der Nierentransplantation bei Kindern. Z. Kinderchir. 1985; 40:260–262.

11 Conley S.B., Flechner S.M., Gilbert R., Van Buren C.T., Brewer E.D., Kahan B.D. Use of Cyclosporine in pediatric renal transplant recipients J. Ped. 1985; 106:45–49

12 Starzl T.E., Iwatsuki S., Malatack J.J., Zitelli B.J., Gartner J.C., Hakala T.R., Rosenthal J.T., Shaw BW. Liver and kidney transplantation in children receiving Cyclosporin A and steroids. J. Ped. 1982; 100:681–686.

13 Bunzendahl H., Offner G., Wonigeit K., Brodehl J., Pichlmayr R. Cyclosporin treatment in pediatric kidney transplantation. In: Paediatric Nephrology. Brodehl J., Erich J.H.H. (eds), Springer Verlag, 1984; pp. 154–157.

14 Tiller D.J., Hall B.M., Horvath J.S., Duggin G.G., Thompson J.F., Sheil A.G.R. Gout and hyperuricaemia in patients on Cyclosporin and diuretics. Lancet 1985; i:453.

15 Thompson C.B., June C.H., Sulivan K.M., Thomas E.D. Association between Cyclosporin neurotoxicity and hypomagnesaemia. Lancet 1984; ii:1116–1120.

16 Knight J.F., Roy L.P., Sheil A.G.R. Catch-up growth in children with successful renal transplants immunosuppressed with Cyclosporin alone. Lancet 1985; i:159–160.

17 Flechner S.M., Conley S.B., Van Buren C.T., Rose G., Kerman R.H., Kahan B.D. Impact of Cyclosporin on renal function and growth in pediatric renal transplant recipients. Transpl. Proc. 1985; 17:1284–1288.

PRIMARY USE OF CICLOSPORIN IN 23 PEDIATRIC KIDNEY GRAFT RECIPIENTS: EARLY RESULTS

J.M. POCHET, Y. PIRSON, J.P. SQUIFFLET, J. JAMART, G.P.J. ALEXANDRE

Renal and Transplantation Units, Cliniques Universitaires St. Luc, avenue Hippocrate 10, 1200 Brussels, Belgium

From March 1983 to July 1985, 23 pediatric renal graft recipients were given CyA as basic immunosuppressive therapy. One year patient and graft survival was respectively 95 and 82%. There was 1 death (from lymphoproliferative disorder) and 3 graft losses (2 from rejection, 1 from recurrent glomerulonephritis) during the first year.

The one-year outcome of the subgroup of 15 children receiving a primary parental graft was compared with that of a previous series of 50 children transplanted with a graft of the same origin but given conventional immunosuppressive therapy. Graft survival was excellent in both groups ($87 \pm 9\%$ in the CyA group and $92 \pm 4\%$ in the conventional group); nevertheless, rejection free survival tended to be higher and the mean number of acute rejection episodes per patient lower in the CyA group than in the conventional group: $47 \pm 13\%$ vs $24 \pm 6\%$ ($0.1 < p < 0.2$) and 0.7 ± 0.3 vs 1.5 ± 0.2 ($0.05 < p < 0.06$), respectively. Incidence of hypertension and mean serum creatinine level tended to be higher in the CyA group than in the conventional group ($55 \pm 15\%$ vs $33 \pm 7\%$ ($p > 0.2$) and 1.27 ± 0.19 mg/dl vs 1.00 ± 0.07 mg/dl ($0.1 < p < 0.2$), respectively).

In conclusion, excellent results in renal transplantation are observed in children given CyA. The main advantage of CyA over conventional therapy is apparently a lower risk of acute rejection, as observed in the subgroup of parental graft recipients, which already had the best prognosis under conventional therapy.

Renal transplantation is the best choice for children in end-stage renal failure [1]. Unfortunately, steroids required for immunosuppression have known detrimental effects, especially on linear growth.

In adult cadaver kidney graft recipients, ciclosporin (CyA) lowers the incidence of acute rejections and thus steroid requirements [2]. With the hope of a similar benefit in our pediatric recipients, we decided in 1983 to introduce CyA as their basic immunosuppressant. We now review our preliminary results in the 23 first CyA treated children.

We have previously shown that in children given conventional (azathioprine) therapy, better results are obtained with parental kidneys than with well-matched

---

Correspondence to: Y. Pirson, Renal and Transplantation units, Cliniques Universitaires St. Luc, Avenue Hippocrate 10, 1200 Brussels, Belgium.

cadaver grafts [3]. Whether CyA also lowers steroid requirements in the privileged subgroup of parental graft recipients, without unacceptable side effects – especially nephrotoxicity – has not yet been demonstrated. In order to answer this question, we compare the outcome of primary parental grafts in children given CyA with that of such grafts in children given conventional therapy.

MATERIALS AND METHODS

From March 1983 to July 1985, 16 male and 7 female children (age: 22 months to 14 years; mean 10.1 years) received their first (19), second (1) or third (3) kidney transplant and were given CyA as their basic immunosuppressive regimen. The graft originated from a well-matched cadaver donor in 6 cases (ABO compatible; mean number of HLA-A,B mismatches: 2; mean number of HLA-DR mismatches:0.7) and from a haplo-identical living related donor in 17 cases (14 ABO compatible and 3 ABO incompatible grafts).

Original nephropathy was chronic interstitial nephritis in 14 cases, chronic glomerulonephritis in 5 cases, Wilms' tumor in 1 case, and of unknown etiology in 3 cases. All patients had received at least 1 blood transfusion prior to transplantation: third party in 21, donor specific in 4 (packed cells in 1 and platelets in the 3 ABO incompatible recipients). Eight patients dit not undergo pretransplant dialysis. Four patients were splenectomized: 1 cadaver recipient prior to transplantation and 3 ABO incompatible recipients (for whom the detailed protocol has been previously reported [4]) at the time of transplantation.

CyA was given intravenously (3 mg/kg) for 24 hours, starting a few hours before transplantation, and then orally (10 mg/kg/day). Dosage was adjusted in order to keep serum creatinine level close to normal and CyA serum trough level (RIA) below 80 ng/ml. Steroids were given as iv methylprednisolone for 6 days (total dose 70 mg/kg) and then as oral prednisolone at a starting dose of 17.5–20 mg/day tapered to 5–7.5 mg/day by 9 months. Nine patients received in addition azathioprine (AZA) (1 mg/kg/day). One cadaver recipient and 14 living related graft recipients received a two-week course of antilymphocyte globulins ((Pressimmun, Behring) 50 mg/kg/day for 3 days followed by 25 mg/kg/day for 11 days) initiated 3 days before (living related recipients) or at the time of transplantation (cadaver recipient).

Among the 23 CyA treated patients, 15 had received a primary haplo-identical living related graft. They were compared to 50 conventionally immunosuppressed children who had received a first haplo-identical living related kidney between July 1971 and June 1983. Characteristics of both groups are summarized in Table I. Major differences between them include a significantly higher percentage of splenectomized (at the time of transplantation) and binephrectomized (one year after transplantation) patients in the conventional group. Prophylactic antilymphocyte globulins (see dosage above) were used in 76 and 80% of patients in the conventional

TABLE I

LIVING RELATED FIRST GRAFT
Characteristics of patients groups

	Conventional (n = 50)	Ciclosporin (n = 15)	
Age (years)	1–14 (mean: 8.6)	1–15 (mean: 9.7)	
Cause of renal failure			
CGN	14	3	
CIN	18	9	
HUS	6	0	
other or unknown	12	3	
No of splenectomized patients at the time of transplantation	41	3	$p<0.001$
No of binephrectomized patients at one year	21/46	0/11	$p<0.02$
No of children given prophylactic ALG	38	12	NS

CGN: chronic glomerulonephritis; CIN: chronic interstitial nephritis;
HUS: hemolytic uremic syndrome;
ALG: antilymphocyte globulin.
NS: not significant.

and in the CyA group, respectively. Maintenance conventional treatment consisted of AZA (1.5–2.5 mg/kg/day) and prednisolone (17.5–40 mg/day tapered to 5–7.5 mg/day by 9–11 months). Six of the CyA treated patients were also given AZA (1 mg/kg/day).

Acute rejection was treated by graft irradiation (150 rads) and intravenous methylprednisolone for 6 days (total dose 70 mg/kg). Antilymphocyte globulin (same dose as for prophylactic use) were routinely added for conventionally treated patients but only in case of corticoresistance for CyA treated patients.

Acute rejection and hypertension were retrospectively defined by the need for appropriate therapy. Date of graft loss was the date of death, of resumption of dialysis or of subsequent retransplantation. Death occurring within 3 months of resumption of dialysis was taken into account for survival analysis.

Statistical differences were evaluated by chi-square test with Yates' continuity correction (frequences) and by Student (continuous variables), Wilcoxon (discrete variables) and Mantel-Haenzel (actuarial survival) tests. Charts were reviewed in March 1986. Data analysis is restricted to the first year after transplantation.

RESULTS

Ciclosporin treated patients (whole group)

Patient survival at 6 and 12 months was respectively 100 and 95%. Only one patient died 9 months after transplantation from a polyclonal lymphoproliferative disorder following EBV primary infection. This primary transplanted patient had not undergone splenectomy and had received neither AZA nor antilymphocyte globulins. Withdrawal of CyA and prednisolone led to accelerated rejection and graft removal, but did not reverse the disease.

Graft survival at 6 and 12 months was respectively 91 and 82%. Three grafts were lost: one (1 month after transplantation) from acute rejection, one (11 months after transplantation) from chronic rejection and one (5 months after transplantation) from recurrent focal and segmental glomerulonephritis with the nephrotic syndrome. None of the ABO incompatible grafts were lost.

Rejection free survival at 6 and 12 months was 48%. Mean number of acute rejection crises per patient was 0.9 at 6 months and 0.8 at 12 months. At 6 and 12 months, serum creatinine averaged 1.20 and 1.31 mg/dl, respectively.

Living related primary graft: one-year outcome according to immunosuppressive regimen (Table II)

Patient survival was excellent in both groups. All CyA treated children were alive whereas three patients of the conventional group died during the first month

TABLE II

LIVING RELATED FIRST GRAFT
One-year outcome according to immunosuppressive regimen

	Conventional (n = 50)	Ciclosporin (n = 15)	
Patient survival	94 ± 3%	100%	$p>0.20$
Graft survival	92 ± 4%	87 ± 9%	$p>0.20$
Rejection free survival	24 ± 6%	47 ± 13%	$0.10<p<0.20$
Mean number of acute rejection/patient	1.5 ± 0.2	0.7 ± 0.3	$0.05<p<0.06$
Mean serum creatinine (mg/dl)	1.00 ± 0.07	1.27 ± 0.19	$0.10<p<0.20$
Incidence of hypertension	33 ± 7%	55 ± 15%	$p>0.20$

Results are expressed as mean ± SE or SEM

post transplantation: 1 from aspiration, 1 from pulmonary oedema (following transplantectomy for recurrent glomerulonephritis) and 1 from sepsis.

Graft survival was identical in both groups. Recurrent glomerulonephritis accounted for 1 graft loss in each group. In the CyA group, one additional graft was lost at one month due to irreversible rejection.

At one year, the rejection free survival tended to be higher and the incidence of acute rejection crises lower in the CyA group than in the conventional group (see Table II). However, the difference did not reach statistical significance. Mean serum creatinine was higher – although not significantly – in the CyA group. The incidence of hypertension in the conventional group as a whole was 33% (46 patients) and 32% in the subgroup of 25 non binephrectomized patients, whereas it reached 55% in the CyA group as a whole (none of them was binephrectomized).

DISCUSSION

Despite the inclusion of some high risk patients (3 third grafts; 3 ABO incompatible grafts) overall results in CyA treated children are most encouraging since 82% of recipients have a functioning graft at one year, without any rejection in nearly two-thirds of them (10/16 patients).

With conventional therapy, such a graft survival rate has already been reached [5,6,7], but in our previously reported study, as early as 3 months after transplantation, only one-third of the surviving grafts remained free of rejection [3].

The only death was due to a polyclonal lymphoproliferative disorder consecutive to EBV primary infection. This case deserves some comments. It is the only one we have observed among our series of more than 200 transplanted patients treated with CyA. The fact that immunosuppressive withdrawal was delayed may explain why, unlike Starzl, we did not observe reversal of the lymphoproliferative disorder [8]. Overt EBV primary infection should perhaps impose a prompt and substantial reduction of immunosuppressive regimen in order to prevent uncontrolled polyclonal lymphoproliferation.

Two grafts were lost due to rejection despite CyA treatment. One acute irreversible rejection occurred despite the prophylactic use of antilymphocyte globulins and a sustained CyA dosage above 10 mg/kg/day. Chronic rejection with eventual graft loss occurred in a high-risk recipient who had previously rejected two other grafts under conventional therapy and was hyperimmunized (lymphocytotoxic antibodies against 83% of the panel). A third graft was lost from recurrent focal and segmental proliferative glomerulonephritis: original glomerulonephritis had presented as steroid-resistant nephrotic syndrome; heavy proteinuria recurred immediately after transplantation and led to graft removal after 5 months. This observation is noteworthy as CyA has recently been advocated for treatment of steroid-resistant nephrotic syndrome [9].

Among living related primary graft recipients, patient and graft survival were as good in CyA as in conventionally treated patients despite the inclusion of 3 ABO incompatible recipients in the CyA group. As we found in adult cadaver kidney recipients [2], the additional advantage of CyA in children receiving a primary parental graft seems to be a reduced – although not significantly – incidence of acute rejection episodes, 47% of the CyA treated children being free of acute rejection at one year vs only 24% of the conventionally treated patients. This observation is especially noteworthy as most conventionally treated patients had undergone splenectomy, a procedure thought to reduce the incidence of early acute rejection [10]. The lower incidence of acute rejection crises allows the cumulative dose of steroids and thus its detrimental effects, especially on linear growth, to be reduced.

Except for the lymphoproliferative syndrome discussed above, no serious side effect of CyA was recorded. As we previously noted in adult cadaver kidney recipients [2], serum creatinine was higher, but not significantly so, in CyA treated children. The higher – although not significant – incidence of hypertension among CyA treated children is not due to the persistance of the native kidney(s), since it is also observed when only non binephrectomized subjects are considered. It is likely related to CyA itself, whose hypertensive effect has been recently demonstrated [11].

In children, the main benefit of CyA over conventional therapy is apparently a lower risk of acute rejection crises. This is observed in the subgroup of primary parental graft recipients, which has already the highest graft survival under conventional treatment in our experience. In this privileged category, selected CyA treated patients might no longer need steroids in the long term [12]. For children in renal failure, kidney transplantation with CyA immunosuppression may be the best chance to achieve optimal growth and development, provided extended follow-up of CyA treated children indicates that the development of chronic rejection is also reduced and that chronic nephrotoxicity is avoided.

ACKNOWLEDGEMENTS

The authors thank Professor van Ypersele de Strihou for his helpful critical advice.

REFERENCES

1 Fine R.N. Renal transplantation for children – the only realistic choice. Kidney Int. 1985; 28:S15–S17.

2 Squifflet J.P., Pirson Y., Jamart J., Wallemacq P., Westelinck K., Alexandre G.P.J. Cyclosporin in cadaver renal transplantation at a center with good results using conventional treatment. Transpl. Proc. 1985; 17:1212–1217.

3 Squifflet J.P., Pirson Y., Van Cangh P., Otte J.B., Van Ypersele de Strihou C., Alexandre G.P.J. Renal transplantation in children: a comparative study between parental and well-matched cadaveric grafts. Transplantation 1981; 32:278–281.

4 Alexandre G.P.J., Squifflet J.P., De Bruyere M., Latinne D., Moriau M., Ikabu N., Carlier M., Pirson Y. Splenectomy as a prerequisite for successful human ABO-incompatible renal transplantation. Transpl. Proc. 1985; 17:138–143.

5 DeShazo C.V., Simmons R.L., Bernstein D.M., DeShazo M.M., Wilmert J., Kjellstrand C.M., Najarian J.S. Results of renal transplantation in 100 children. Surgery 1974; 76:461–468.
6 Novick A.C., Karamooz M., Braun W.E., Steinmuller D. Results of renal transplantation in children. J. Urol. 1980; 124:787–789.
7 Squifflet J.P., Pirson Y., Jamart J., Alexandre G.P.J. Hundred renal transplantations in children. Eur. J. Pediat. 1983; 140:190.
8 Starzl T.E., Nalesnik M.A., Porter K.A., Ho M., Bahnson H.T. Reversibility of lymphomas and lymphoproliferative lesions developing under cyclosporin-steroid therapy. Lancet 1984; i:583–588.
9 Meyrier A., Simon P., Perret G., Condamin-Meyrier M.C. Remission of idiopathic nephrotic syndrome after treatment with cyclosporin A. Br. Med. J. 1986; 292:789–792.
10 Kauffman H.M., Swanson M.K., McGregor W.R., Rodgers R.E., Fox P.S. Splenectomy in renal transplantation Surg. Gynecol. Obstet. 1974; 139:33–40.
11 De Plaen J.F., Ferrant A., Uten M., Uyttebrouck A., Michaux J.L., Van Ypersele de Strihou C. Cyclosporin A induced hypertension in bone marrow transplantation. Kidney Int. 1985; 28:394.
12 Flechner S.M., Kerman R.H., Van Buren C.T., Epps L., Kahan B.D. The use of cyclosporin in living-related renal transplantation. Transplantation 1984; 38:685–691.

USE OF CICLOSPORIN FOR MAINTENANCE IMMUNOSUPPRESSION FOLLOWING PEDIATRIC RENAL TRANSPLANTATION

D.F. GEARY, R. BAUMAL, G.S. ARBUS

Department of Pediatrics (Nephrology) and Pathology, The Hospital for Sick Children, Toronto, Ontario, Canada.

CyA has been used as a maintenance immunosuppressive agent in 18 children following renal transplantation at The Hospital for Sick Children, Toronto. Five high-risk patients received CyA 5-10 mg/kg/day prior to December 1984. Two of these died of treatment-related causes. Azathioprine was substituted for CyA in the other 3 children, 2-4 months post-transplantation. Following this change in therapy, 1 patient developed an acute rejection episode. Between December 1984 and October 1985, 13 children received a lower dose of CyA together with prednisone and azathioprine. Four of these grafts have failed – 2 due to rejection.

Our observations do not permit absolute conclusions to be drawn. Nonetheless, we recommend the use of low-dose CyA as part of maintenance immunosuppression for pediatric renal transplant recipients, once urine output has been established.

The value of ciclosporin (CyA) for maintenance immunosuppression following renal transplantation has been clearly demonstrated in controlled clinical trials in adults [1,2]. Little information is available on the use of CyA in children, although preliminary reports appear to confirm its value. Because of uncertainty concerning the long-term side effects of CyA, it was initially recommended at our institution for maintenance immunosuppression only in selected high risk patients. More recently however, based on our experience using CyA to treat chronic renal transplant rejection, a lower dose of CyA has been employed for maintenance immunosuppression, in the majority of transplant recipients. This report describes our experience in 18 children treated with CyA from the time of transplantation, between July 1983 and October 1985.

METHODS

All patients were transplanted and subsequently followed at the Renal Transplant Clinic of The Hospital for Sick Children, Toronto. Each child received at least

Correspondence to: D.F. Geary, Division of Nephrology, Department of Pediatrics, The Hospital for Sick Children, 555 University Avenue, Toronto, Ontario, Canada M5G 1XB

5 blood transfusions prior to transplantation, and all were recipients of cadaveric grafts. There were 9 girls and 9 boys, aged between 1.0 - 18.0 years at the time of transplantation. The patients have been arbitrarily divided into 2 groups – Group A being those transplanted prior to December 1984, and Group B, patients who were transplanted after this date.

There were 5 patients in Group A, all of whom were considered at high risk because they had aggressively rejected previous transplants, and in 2 of whom it was hoped that the steroid sparing effect of CyA might enhance their growth. Their ages ranged from 7.5 – 18.0 years. All were loaded with CyA 15 mg/kg, I.V. preoperatively, and this was subsequently changed to the oral route at a dose of 5 – 10 mg/kg/day to maintain trough serum CyA levels between 80-200 ng/ml. These patients received prednisone as their only other maintenance immunosuppressive agent.

The patients in Group B have all been transplanted since December 1984 and represent 13 of the total 20 transplants performed during that time. These children varied in age from 1.0-17.5 years, and 7 were first graft recipients. All of these patients received rabbit antithymocyte serum or horse antilymphocyte globulin for the first 7-14 days post-transplantation after which CyA 3-6 mg/kg/day was prescribed if satisfactory urine output and renal function were established. Trough serum CyA levels were maintained between 20-120 ng/ml. Each of these patients was also prescribed maintenance prednisone and azathioprine (AZA).

Side effects were attributed to CyA treatment if they had been previously described, and were observed in our patients. A distinction between adverse effects due to CyA and side effects due to other drugs and problems associated with transplant rejection could not always be made with certainty.

RESULTS

The original disease causing renal failure in each group of patients is listed in Table 1. It is noteworthy that 1 patient in each group originally developed renal failure as a consequence of hemolytic uremic syndrome.

The outcome for all patients treated with CyA and their length of follow-up is shown in Table 2. The mean daily CyA dose used to treat patients in Group A was 8.0 mg/kg/day and that in Group B was 5.4 mg/kg/day. It had been planned to discontinue CyA after 3 months in the surviving patients in Group A and this was carried out in 2; because of an episode of suspected CyA nephrotoxicity, it was stopped after 2 months in the third child. AZA was substituted for CyA in these children. The mean serum creatinine values for these patients at the time CyA was discontinued was 92 $\pm$ 82 μmol/l. Following cessation of CyA and substitution of AZA, 1 patient maintains stable renal function, a second developed chronic rejection and the third has undergone an episode of steroid responsive rejection with some residual impairment of renal function. The 2 deaths in Group

Table I

Original disease causing renal failure

	Group A	Group B
Dysplasia/Hypoplasia	0	2
Focal Sclerosis	2	4
Membranoproliferative GN	2	0
Congenital Nephrosis	0	3
Hemolytic Uremic Syndrome	1	1
Other	0	3

Table II

Follow-up of patients treated with CyA

	Group A (n = 5)	Group B (n = 13)	
Follow-up (yr)	1.46 ± 0.62	0.28 ± 0.21	(x ± SD)
Creatinine (μmol/l)	172 ± 57	110 ± 46	(x ± SD)
Dose CyA (mg/kg/day)	8.0	5.4	
Graft Loss	0	4	
Died	2	0	

A resulted from a disseminated cytomegalovirus infection in 1 patient, and following the sudden and unexpected development of acute pulmonary edema in the other.

Four patients in Group B have lost their grafts. Two transplants failed due to uncontrollable rejection, which in 1 case, followed withdrawal of CyA because of acute nephrotoxicity. Although rejection also contributed to the other 2 graft failures, other factors may also have been involved. As shown in Table 3, a large number of patients have side effects attributed to CyA although CyA may not have been solely responsible in each case. Hypertension, for example, may have resulted from fluid overload, steroids, or graft rejection, although it is noteworthy that hypertension was also observed in otherwise healthy patients with normal renal function.

DISCUSSION

In Group A patients, the dose of CyA prescribed was similar to that in most published studies of both adults and children. Although rejection did not occur in this group, nephrotoxicity was observed in 2 patients, while 2 others died of causes which were probably treatment related. Resuscitation of the child who developed acute pulmonary edema following discharge from our institution, was

Table III

Number of patients exhibiting side effects attributable to CyA (n = 18).

Nephrotoxicity	-Acute	4
	-Chronic	2
Hyperkalemia		3
Hypertension		18
Hirsutism		10
Thrombotic		1
Infection		6

attempted at the local hospital without success. Permission for autopsy was refused. It is suspected that this death resulted from a coronary artery thrombosis; an increased incidence of thromboembolic complications has been described in transplant patients treated with CyA[5]. AZA was electively substituted for CyA in 3 patients of Group A within a few months of transplantation. The changeover was uneventful in 2 children in whom the prednisone dose was temporarily increased, but in the third child whom the steroid dose was unaltered, an acute rejection episode developed. This suggests that conversion from CyA to azathioprine can be successfully achieved; the development of frequent acute rejection episodes which have been previously described [6,7] may be avoided if the daily maintenance prednisone dose is temporarily increased at the time of changeover.

Toward the end of 1984, the immunosuppression policy in renal transplants at The Hospital for Sick Children was changed. This was based in part, on the experience of the Canadian multicentre study [1] which showed poorer graft survival in CyA treated patients if the donor kidney was stored by machine perfusion for longer than 24 hours. Since many of our patients undergoing transplantation must be flown to Toronto from across Canada, necessitating surgical delays, it was decided that CyA should no longer be introduced at the time of transplantation, but rather 1-2 weeks later. Also, based on experience gained in treating patients with chronic renal transplant rejection, the recommended dose of CyA was reduced to 3-5 mg/kg/day.

Four grafts have been lost in Group B patients since the introduction of this new immunosuppression policy. Two of these failures resulted from biopsy-proven rejection, in 1 of whom the graft was lost after acute nephrotoxicity necessitated withdrawal of CyA. The cause of graft loss in the other 2 children is uncertain. In 1, the renal biopsy showed marked hyalinosis of the vessel walls which was thought to have resulted from renal ischemia, with only mild vascular rejection (Figure), although renal function had been excellent in the first few post-operative days. The remaining graft failure was associated with Pseudomonas septicemia in a young child, the donor for whom was less than 1 year old. As we have previously

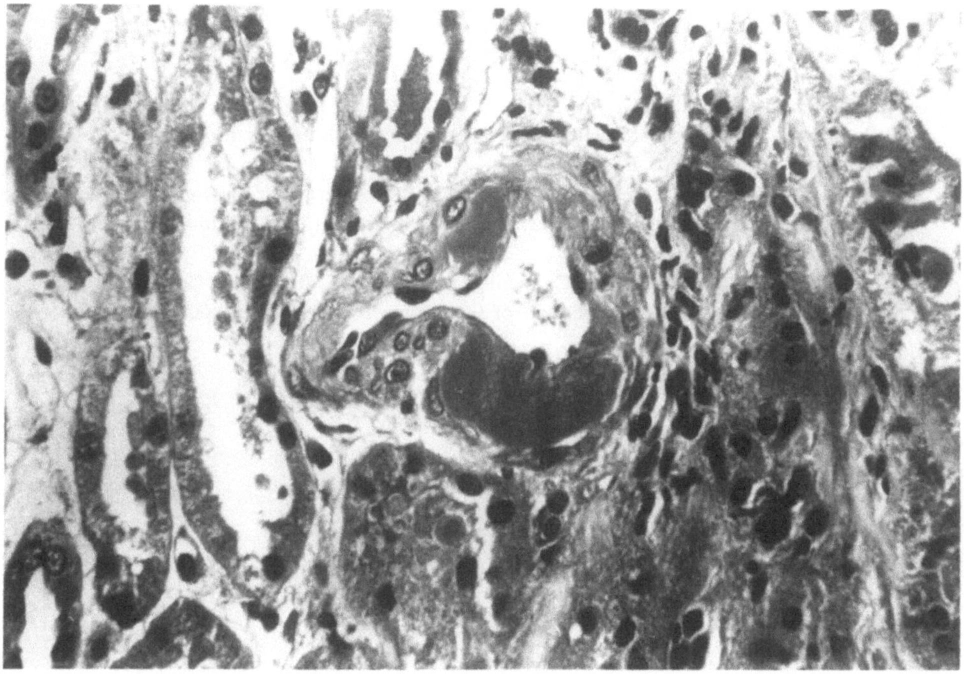

Hyalinosis in vessel wall attributed to renal ischemia.

reported, the results of transplantation at our institution using such young donors are seldom satisfactory and the cause of graft loss is often difficult to precisely define [8].

We feel therefore that although absolute conclusions cannot be drawn after such a short follow-up period, our results justify the use of low-dose CyA for pediatric renal transplant recipients. However, we do not recommend its introduction until urine output is clearly established and renal function is satisfactory. In the immediate post-operative period, a course of antilymphocyte globulin is recommended until such time as CyA can be safely introduced.

REFERENCES

1 The Canadian Multicentre Transplant Study Group. A randomized clinical trial of Cyclosporine in cadaveric renal transplantation. N. Engl. J .Med. 1983; 309: 809-815.

2 European Multicentre Trial Group. Cyclosporin in cadaveric renal transplantation: One year follow-up of a multicentre trial. Lancet 1983; ii:986–989.

3 Hoyer P.F., Offner G., Wonigeit K., Brodehl J., Pichelmayr R. Dosage of Cyclosporine A in children with renal transplants. Clin. Nephrol. 1984; 22:68–71.

4 Conley S.B., Flechner S.M., Gilbert R., Van Buren C.T., Brewer E.D., Kahan B.D. Use of Cyclosporine in pediatric renal transplant recipients J. Ped. 1985; 106:45–49.

5 Vanrenterghem Y., Lerut T., Roels L., Gruwez J., Michielsen P., Gresele P., Colucci M., Deckmyn H., Arnout J., Vermylen J., Thromboembolic complications and haemostatic changes in Cyclosporin-treated cadaveric kidney allograft recipients. Lancet 1985; i:999–1002.

6 Vanrenterghem Y., Waer M., Michielsen P. A controlled trial of one versus three months Cyclosporine and conversion to azathioprine in renal transplantation. Transpl. Proc. 1985; 17:1162–1163.

7 Wood R.F.M., Thompson J.F., Ting A., Benjamin I.S., Allen N.H., Morris P.J. A randomized controlled trial of short term Cyclosporine therapy in renal transplantation (Trial II). Transpl. Proc. 1985; 17:1164–1165.

8 Arbus G.S., Hardy B.E., Balfe J.W., Churchill B.M., Steele B.T., Baumal R., Curtis R.N. Cadaveric renal transplants in children under 6 years of age. Kidney Int. 1983; 24 (suppl. 15):S111–S115.

MANAGEMENT OF KIDNEY TRANSPLANTATION WITH CICLOSPORIN: CLINICAL EXPERIENCE IN 43 CHILDREN.

G. OFFNER, P.F. HOYER, H.P. KROHN, H. JUEPPNER, J. BRODEHL

Department of Pediatric Nephrology, Medical School Hannover, P.O. Box 610180, D-3000 Hannover 61, Federal Republic of Germany

Experience with CyA after kidney transplantation in children is presented. The survival rate for patients and grafts is considerably higher after two and 3 years than with conventional immunosuppression with AZA and high doses of steroids. There was a high frequency of acute reversible rejection episodes within the first month.

Due to the potent immunosuppressive properties of ciclosporin (CyA), the dose of prednisolone required for optimal immunosuppression is considerably lower than with conventional therapy. It was, therefore, expected that especially children with uremic growth retardation would benefit from CyA. In the following, pediatric experience with the new immunosuppressive drug is presented.

PATIENTS AND METHODS

From September 1982 to November 1985, 43 children were treated with CyA from the time they received a kidney transplant. One child with hyperoxaluria was excluded. There were 21 boys and 22 girls, 8 received living related kidneys and 35 cadaveric kidneys. 39 children got the first graft, 1 child a second and 3 children a third graft. Their chronological age at time of transplantation ranged between 2–16 years, their bone age between 2 and 15 years (Table I).

The original diseases, leading to endstage renal failure, are depicted in Table II. 63% of the patients had a congenital renal disease, these included renal dysplasia (8), nephronophthisis (6), cystinosis (6), obstructive uropathy (6) and infantile cystic kidneys (1). The remaining 37% suffered from an acquired disease: hemolytic uremic syndrome (3), focal sclerosis (4), reflux nephropathies (4), and proliferative glomerulonephritis (3). Miscellaneous disease represents one child with hypersensitive angiitis and one child with IgA nephritis.

The quality of the donor kidneys in the 43 recipients is summarized in Table III. The

Correspondence to: G. Offner, Department of Pediatric Nephrology, Medical School Hannover, P.O. Box 610180, D-3000 Hannover 61, Federal Republic of Germany.

TABLE I

Pediatric kidney transplantation with CyA

	boys N = 21	girls N = 22	total N = 43
LRD/CD	3/18	5/17	8/35
first graft	18	21	39
second graft	1	-	1
third graft	2	1	3
chronol. age at Tx range in yrs	2–16	5–16	2–16
Bone age at Tx range in yrs	2–14.5	2–15	2–15

TABLE II

Original diseases of children with kidney transplantation

Congenital/familial	27 = 63%	Acquired	16 = 37%
Dys-/Hypoplasia	8	Hem. urem. S.	3
Nephronophthisis	6	Focal sclerosis	4
Cystinosis	6	Reflux nephropathy	4
Obst.Uropathy	6	Prol. GN	3
Miscellaneous	1	Miscellaneous	2

TABLE III

Pediatric kidney transplantation with CyA (n = 43)

primary function	36 = 84%
cold ischemia time (hrs)	20.3
range	0–40
4 HLA miss-matches	7 = 16%
4 HLA identical matches	1 = 2%
living related donors	8 = 19%

mean cold ischemia time was 20.3 hrs with a range between 0-40 hrs. Seven kidneys (16%) revealed a total mismatch, and 1 was HLA-identical. The 8 living related kidneys were one-haploidentical. Under routine volume expansion post transplantation, 36 kidneys (84%) had a good function within the first 24 hours.

The immunosuppressive therapy was started 6 hrs prior to transplantation with a single oral dose of 500 mg CyA/m^2 body surface area. Within 6 hrs postoperatively the same amount of CyA was to be given in two doses. After 1 week CyA dose was reduced weekly by 50 mg/m^2/day. Whole blood concentration of CyA was determined twice per week using the commercially available Sandoz RIA kit. The desired therapeutic range as determined by trough whole blood levels was considered to be 200 to 750 ng/ml. Prednisolone was administered intraoperatively in a dose of 300 mg/m^2 followed by 60 mg/m^2/day during the first and 30 mg/m^2/day during the second week post transplantation. Prednisolone was subsequently reduced weekly to a final dose of 4 mg/m^2/day after 7 weeks (Table IV).

TABLE IV

Immunosuppressive regimen with ciclosporin and low dose prednisolone

Time	Ciclosporin Dosage (mg/m^2/day p.o.)	Prednisolone Dosage (mg/m^2/day)
6 hours preoperative	500	-
intraoperative	-	300
Week 1	500*	60*
Week 2	450*	30**
Week 3	400*	15**
Week 4	350*	12**
Week 5	300*	9**
Week 6	300*	6**
Week 7 and thereafter	300*	4**

Target range for CyA-trough blood concentrations 200–750 ng/ml
* Administered in two doses per day
** Administered in a single dose per day
Treatment of acute rejection episodes: Prednisolone (for 3– 6 days) 300–900 mg/m^2/day i.v.

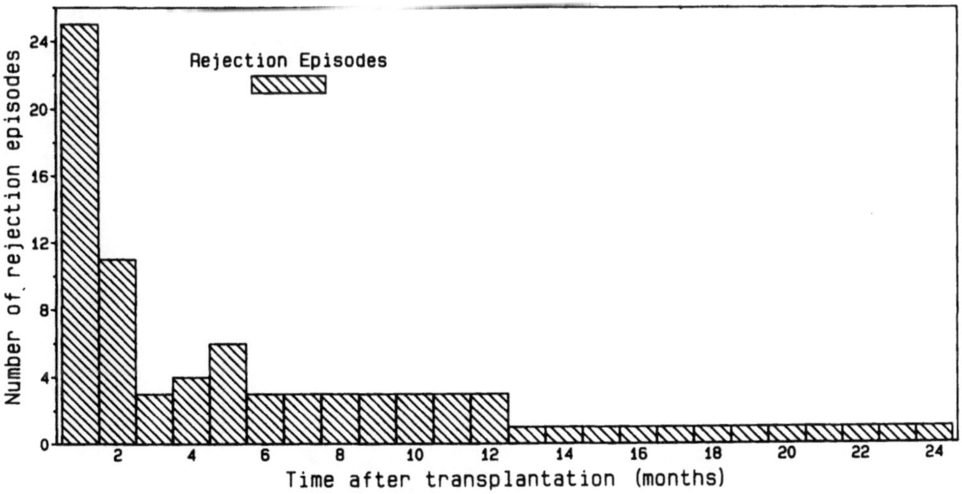

Fig. 1. The frequency of acute rejection episodes per month following 43 pediatric kidney transplantations with CyA.

RESULTS

Acute rejection episodes occurred with the highest frequency during the first month in which 25 episodes were observed. 12 rejections were observed during the second month, thereafter only 1–3 rejections per month (Fig. 1).

Table V summarizes the number of rejection episodes per patient per year in relation to the observed patients and the percentage of rejecting patients. During the first year 69% of the recipients suffered from acute rejections with a mean frequency of 2.0 per patient. Half of the rejection occurred during the first month. During the second year only 19 patients had a transplant rejection with a mean rate of 0.8 per patient. In the third year, which only 5 children completed so far, no rejection episode was observed.

TABLE V

Acute rejections in pediatric kidney transplantation with CyA

Period	Rej/pat	Observed pat	Rejecting pat %
1st year	2.0	32	69
2nd year	0.8	19	37
3rd year	0	5	0

The actuarial survival rate for both patients and grafts, is 97% after 1 year (Fig. 2.). One child died from klebsiella sepsis 5 months after transplantation with a functioning graft. After two years patient survival remained 97%, graft survival decreased to 93% because one patient experienced severe rejection episodes and had to go back on dialysis. So far only 5 patients have completed 3 years. Survival rate is reduced to 85%, patient survival rate remains unchanged.

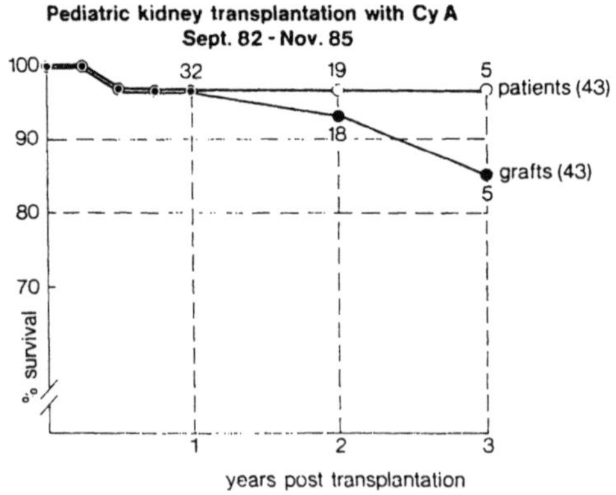

Fig. 2. Survival rates of 43 children and grafts following kidney transplantation with CyA.

EXPERIENCE OF CICLOSPORIN USE IN THE FIRST THREE MONTHS AFTER KIDNEY TRANSPLANTATION IN PEDIATRIC PATIENTS. A PRELIMINARY REPORT

MARIA C.J.W. DE JONG[1], LEO A.H. MONNENS[1], ANDRIES J. HOITSMA[2]

[1]Department of Pediatrics, [2]Department of Medicine, Division of Nephrology, St. Radboud Ziekenhuis, Nijmegen, The Netherlands.

Preliminary results of CyA treatment during the first three months following kidney transplantation in 11 children are reported. CyA was given combined with a low dose of Prednisone. Three months after transplantation all patients were converted to AZA. Six patients experienced 7 reversible rejection episodes within the first three months. Three patients experienced 3 reversible rejection episodes within 3 weeks of conversion to AZA. Three patients had no rejection (follow-up 26–22–12 months). Graft survival rate at three months was 100%, at 6 months and 1 year 89%.

At this moment it is not statistically significant that children, treated with CyA have less rejection episodes, but it is at least striking that of 34 AZA treated children all but one experienced a rejection episode within 3 months after transplantation and of 11 CyA treated children 3 didn't have a rejection episode.

Ciclosporin (CyA) is more and more used as immunosuppressive agent, with or without prednison, in kidney transplantation [1], also in children.[2,3,4] In our hospital about 80 kidney transplantations are performed every year, ± 10% of them are children. Looking for the best immunosuppressive treatment, a prospective trial was started in October 1983. A total number of 200 patients will be studied. By lot, half of the patients receive Azathioprine (AZA) and Prednisone; the other half CyA and low dose Prednisone during the first 3 months. Our report concerning the children, is still preliminary.

PATIENTS AND METHODS

Between August 1977 and September 1985 39 children received 45 kidney grafts. Their age varied between 4 and 18.2 years, with a mean age of 11.9 years. Two children received a graft from a parental donor; 37 children received 43 cadaveric grafts. Between 1979 and 1983 all patients received one transfusion with leucocyte

Correspondence to: M.C.J.W. de Jong, Department of Pediatrics, St. Radboud Ziekenhuis, Geert Grooteplein Zuid 20, 6500 HB Nijmegen, The Netherlands poor blood. From 1983 all patients received one to three transfusions with fresh packed cells without buffy coat. Before October 1983 all patients were treated with AZA and Prednisone. Since October 1983 the children participated in the prospective trial. Until September 1985 11 children were treated with CyA and low dose Prednisone; 5 children with AZA and Prednisone. CyA is only used in the first three months after transplantation [5]. The treatment regimen is presented in Table I. After three months CyA is converted to AZA. Prednisone was increased to 25 mg/1.73 m^2/day for one week in the first patients, and than back to the maintenance dose; now it is increased to 25 mg/1.73 m^2/day for one week and than tapered in about 6 weeks to the maintenance dose.

A first rejection episode is treated by anti-thymocyte globulin; a second rejection by high doses of Prednisone orally. A renal biopsy was always performed upon suspicion of a second rejection.

Until December 1985 11 children were treated with CyA and converted to Aza. Their mean age was 10.7 years (range 5.1–17.2 years). All received a cadaveric graft. For two children it was a second graft. CyA levels were assayed in heparinized whole blood.

RESULTS

In table II the following data of the 11 patients are summarized: age, sex, primary disease, date of transplant, HLA A–B–DR mismatches, transplantnumber, episodes

TABLE I

Treatment regimen in the Ciclosporin group

Ciclosporin
Six hours after transplantation for a minimum of 48 hrs and a maximum of 72 hrs
3 mg/kg/24 hours i.v.

Day 3 – day 14	17.5 mg/kg/24 hours	in 3 doses p.o
Wk 3 – wk 5	13.5 "	"
Wk 5 – wk 7	11.5 "	"
Wk 7 – wk 9	9.5 "	"
Wk 9 – wk 11	7.5 "	"
Wk 11 – wk 13	5.5 "	"

Prednisone

Pretransplant	100 mg Prednisolone/ 1.73 m^2	i.v.			
Day 1	"	"			in 4 doses
Day 2	100 mg/ 1.73 m^2	p.o.	in	4	doses
Day 3	25 mg/ "	"	in	2	doses
Day 4	20 mg/ "	"	"		
Day 5	15 mg/ "	"	"		
Day 6	10 mg/ "	"	"		(is maintenance dose)

TABLE II

Data of 11 CyA treated patients

Case nr.	Age (y) Sex	Primary disease	Date of transplant	number of HLA mismatches A B	number of HLA mismatches D R	Transplant number	Outcome 1 Dec. 1985 rejection episodes hypertension medication function
1	17.2 M	Reflux N.	15-10-83	2	1	2	no rejection no hypertension P 0.17 mg/kg Daily AZA 2.8 mg/kg Serum creat. 90 μmol/l.
2	15 M	Urethral. valves	22-10-83	2	0	2	1 rejection day 97 hypertension P 0.17 mg/kg Daily AZA 2.5 mg/kg Serum creat. 129 μmol/l.
3	11.6 F	Nephro-nophthisis	17-02-84	2	1	1	no rejection hypertension P 0.15 mg/kg Alternate days AZA 2.3 mg/kg Serum creat. 59 μmol/l.
4	5.2 F	Focal glom. sclerose	06-04-84	2	0	1	2 rejections day 60/180 hypertension P 0.28 mg/kg Alternate days AZA 2.8 mg/kg Serum creat. 216 μmol/l.
5	9.8 F	Reflux N.	19-05-84	2	0	1	2 rejections day 30/150 no hypertension P 0,24 mg/kg Alternate days AZA 2 mg/kg Serum creat. 62 μmol/l.
6	10.5 M	Urethral. valves	23-12-84	3	1	1	no rejection no hypertension P 0,24 mg/kg Daily AZA 2,4 mg/kg Serum creat. 102 μmol/l.
7	6,6 M	Extra-capil. GN	06-01-85	4	1	1	2 rejections day 13/43 hypertension died 16-05-85 decompensatio cordis serum creat. 112 μmol/l.
8	8.9	Dysplasia	21-01-85	3	0	1	3 rejections day 20/90/135 hypertension P 0.27 mg/kg Alternate days Cyclo 5.3 mg/kg Serum creat. 154 μmol/l.
9	7.8 M	Congenital nefrot.S.	19-05-85	2	1	1	2 rejections day 75/150 hypertension P 0.31 mg/kg Daily AZA 2.3 mg/kg Serum creat. 139 μmol/l
10	13.9 M	Nephro-nophthisis	19-06-85	1	0	1	1 rejection day 105 no hypertension P 0.27 mg/kg Daily AZA 2.7 mg/kg Serum creat. 93 μmol/l
11	12.2 M	H.U.S.	16-08-85	2	1	1	1 rejection day 22 no hypertension P 0.5 mg/kg Daily AZA 2.6 mg/kg Serum creat. 61 μmol/l

of rejection, immunosuppressive therapy, serum creatinine and presence of hypertension on the first of December 1985. By comparing 11 CyA treated children with 34 AZA treated children, there is at three months only a statistically significant difference in serum creatinine level (97±19.8 μmol/l. in the CyA group vs 75±18.9 μmol/l. in the AZA group). Concerning proteinuria, hypertension, number of rejections, no statistically significant difference is present. One year after transplantation the difference in serum creatinine has disappeared (96±36 μmol/l. in CyA group vs 120±86 μmol/l. in the AZA group). Although there is no statistically significant difference in the frequency of rejection, it is striking that in the AZA group all but one of the 34 patients experienced a rejection within the first three months after transplantation, while in the CyA group 3 out of 11 patients had no rejection episode with a follow-up of 26, 22 and 10 months respectively (Table III).

TABLE III

Frequency of rejection

	N	Rejection frequency		
Group without Ciclosporin	30	0		1 patient
		1		14 patients
		2		8 "
		3		7 "
Total amount of rejection episodes			51	
Group with 3 months Ciclosporin	11	0		3 patients
		1		4 "
		2		3 "
		3		1 "
Total amount of rejection episodes			13	

TABLE IV

Treatment regimen in Azathioprine group

Azathioprine			
pretransplantation	3 mg/kg	i.v.	
posttransplantation	3 mg/kg/day	p.o.	
Prednisone			
pretransplantation	100 mg/1.73 m²	i.v.	
day 1	100 mg/1.73 m²/day	i.v.	in 4 divided doses
day 2	100 mg/1.73 m²/day	p.o.	in 4 divided doses
day 3– 30	25 mg/1.73 m²/day	p.o.	in 2 divided doses
day 30–100	20 mg/1.73 m²/day	p.o.	in 2 divided doses
> day 100	tapering to 10 mg/1.73 m²/day		

DISCUSSION

The limited number of studied children allows only some preliminary conclusions. As generally observed the serum creatinine level after 3 months of CyA treatment was higher than in the group treated with AZA [6]. Nine months later this difference has disappeared. All children developed some degree of hirsutism and hyperkalemia [7]. Sometimes a slight tremor became evident. It is clear that during CyA treatment less Prednisone was required than during AZA treatment (Table IV). Our hope is that CyA treatment will diminish the number of rejections and infectious complications after transplantation. This will permit the use of a lower dose of Prednisone and in this way, a better growth of the children [8,9,10].

REFERENCES

1 Salaman J.R. Cyclosporin in renal transplantation: a guide to management. Lancet 1984; ii:269–271.
2 Hoyer P.F., Offner G., Wonigeit K., Brodehl J., Pichelmayr R. Dosage of Cyclosporine A in children with renal transplants. Clin. Nephrol. 1984; 22:68–71.
3 Conley S.B., Flechner S.M., Gilbert R., Van Buren C.T., Brewer E.D., Kahan B.D. Use of Cyclosporine in pediatric renal transplant recipients J. Ped. 1985; 106:45–49.
4 Brodehl J., Pichelmayr R., Offner G. 14 Jahre Nierentransplantation bei Kindern. Monatsschr. Kinderheilk. 1985; 133:771–773.
5 Morris P.J., French M.E., Dunnill M.S., Hunnisett A.G.W., Ting A., Thompson J.F., Wood R.F.M. A controlled trial of Cyclosporine in renal transplantation with conversion to azathioprine and prednisolone after three months. Transplantation 1983; 36:273–277.
6 Chapman J.R., Harding N.G.L., Griffiths D., Morris P.J. Reversibility of Cyclosporin nephrotoxicity after three months' treatment. Lancet 1985; i:128–129.
7 Foley R.J., Hammer R.W., Weinman E.J. Serum potassium concentrations in Cyclosporin and azathioprine treated renal transplant patients. Nephron. 1985; 40:280–285.
8 Knight J.F., Roy L.P., Sheil A.G.R. Catch-up growth in children with successful renal transplants immunosuppressed with Cyclosporin alone. Lancet 1985; i:159–160.
9 Klare B., Von Walter J., Hahn H., Emmrich P., Land W. Cyclosporin in renal transplantation in children. Lancet 1984; ii:692.
10 Ellis D., Avner E.D., Rosenthal J.T., Taylor R.J., Young L.W., Palumbi M.A., Hakala T.R. Renal function and somatic growth in pediatric cadaveric renal transplantation with Cyclosporin-prednison immunosuppression. Am. J. Dis. Childh. 1985; 139:1161–1167.

CICLOSPORIN USE IN PEDIATRIC RENAL TRANSPLANTATION : EXPERIENCE WITH 50 PATIENTS

MARIE-FRANCE GAGNADOUX*, GENEVIEVE GUEST*, PATRICK NIAUDET*, CORINNE ANTIGNAC*, FRANÇOIS LOKIEC***, NICOLE HINGLAIS**, MICHEL BROYER*

** Pediatric Nephrology Dept Hôpital des Enfants-Malades, Paris, France, ** I.N.S.E.R.M. U. 192 Hôpital des Enfants-Malades, Paris, France, *** Pharmacology Dept Centre René Huguenin – 92211 Saint-Cloud*

CyA was used in 50 children with renal allografts. The mean CyA dose was 6–8 mg/kg/day. 17 children were electively converted to CyA between the 3rd and the 8th week, either in a randomized protocol starting on 01/01/85, or for non-immunological reasons (mainly cytopenia). 16 grafts are now functioning, but follow-up is less than one year for 15 of them. In the randomized protocol, there is no difference either in the graft survival rate, or in the number of rejection episodes, between the CyA group and the control group treated by prednisone and AZA. Mean creatininemia level is higher (118 μMol/L) in CyA treated patients than in the control group (97 μMol/L). In patients converted to CyA for steroid-resistant rejection, the results are encouraging in early crises (within 1st month) with 66% of normally functioning grafts. On the contrary, the results are poor in later crises (15% of normally functioning grafts). Graft survival rate is excellent in patients converted to CyA for non-immunological reasons. The most worrying side-effects were hypertension and nephrotoxicity, but renal biopsies never showed severe CyA-related lesions.

Ciclosporin (CyA) use in renal transplantation started in our pediatric unit in November 1983 (except for one case, briefly treated in November 1982). The first indications were children with rejection episodes and contra-indication to high doses of corticosteroids. Over the year 1984, we progressively extended the indications to azathioprine (AZA) intolerance and to steroid-resistant rejections. Then, following the report of Soulillou et al who used CyA after two months of conventional therapy with excellent results [1], we decided to give CyA routinely, starting one month after transplantation because of the high incidence of initial anuria in our patients. In order to assess if CyA really adds a beneficial effect, we also chose to compare it with conventional treatment in a randomized trial which started in January 1985. The preliminary results of the first 12 patients included in this trial, as well as the results in the other 38 children treated with CyA in the past two years, are reported here.

Correspondence to: M-F Gagnadoux, Pediatric Nehrology Department, Hôp. Enfants Malades, 75743 Cedex 15, Paris, France.

PATIENTS

From November 1982 to October 1985, among 174 children who received a kidney graft, 50 (49 of them having been treated from November 1983) were treated by CyA. They were 2½ to 19 years old at time of transplantation (mean age: 12½ years), 3 to 21 years old at time of treatment. There were 38 boys and 12 girls.

A – *"Primary use"*

18 patients may be considered in this category:

1 – *Initial use*

Only one patient (second graft with cadaver kidney) received CyA from day 1, because of a supposed psychiatric contra-indication to corticosteroids.

2 – *Early conversion*

Seventeen patients were electively converted to CyA during the first 2 months; 12 of them were included in a randomized protocol starting on 01/01/85 and received CyA from the 2nd month after transplantation; 5 others were converted to CyA between day 23 and day 60 for leukopenia or thrombopenia preventing AZA use (4 cases), and recurrent nephrosis (1 case). Among these 17 patients, there were 16 grafts from cadàver donors, and 1 from living donor; 5 were second grafts.

B – *"Secondary use"*

Thirty-two patients are included in this group. They were converted to CyA between the 15th day and the 11th year for various reasons:

1 – *Steroid-resistant rejection*

Twenty-one patients (19 cadaver kidneys, 2 living donoors; 18 first grafts and 3 second grafts) were converted to CyA for steroid-resistant rejection: 9 during the first month of tranplantation, 8 between 1 and 3 months, and 4 after 6 months.

2 – *Other causes*

Three patients (3 cadaver kidneys, 2 first grafts and one second graft) were converted to CyA (at 2, 2 and 23 months) because of the conjunction of acute

rejection and contra-indication to steroids increase (2 cases) or AZA use (1 case).
Eight additional patients (all cadaver kidneys and first grafts) were converted to CyA after the 6th month for non-immunological reasons: leukopenia or thrombopenia (6 cases), psychiatric indication to decrease steroids (1 case), recurrent nephrosis (1 case).

METHODS

I - *Treatment protocol*

A - *Before January 1985*

The conventional treatment combined AZA (3 mg/kg/day for a GFR > 50 ml/min/1.73m^2) from day 0, and prednisone from day 1 : 60 mg/m^2, tapered to 15 mg/m^2 at 2 months, 9 mg/m^2 at 6 months, 7.5 mg/m^2 at 12 months, and 15 mg/m^2 every other day at 18 months if renal biopsy allowed alternate-day steroid therapy. Antilymphocyte (ALG) or antithymocyte globulin (ATG) were given in case of rejection in some patients.

Except for the first patient, treated in 1982 with 15 mg/kg/day, all patients converted to CyA from 1983 received initial doses not higher than 8 mg/kg/day, and dosage was afterwards adjusted according to plasma levels (see below). They all received low doses of prednisone (7 mg/m^2/day as minimal dosage); AZA was stopped in all patients with hematological toxicity and in most of the others.

B - *From January 1985*

The conventional treatment during the first month included prednisone, AZA, and preventive use of ALG for 2 to 3 weeks after transplantation. At day 30, patients were randomly allocated to triple therapy with prednisone and low dose CyA and AZA, or to conventional treatment with prednisone and AZA.

For patients receiving CyA, the initial dosage was 6 mg/kg/day in 3 divided doses (every 8 hours); the dosage was later adjusted on weekly CyA plasma level in order to obtain a trough level of 50-150 ng/ml and a peak level not higher than 250 ng/ml.

The actual dosage in the 16 children so treated was the following: 1 child received 4 mg/kg/day, 8 received 5 to 7.5 mg/kg/day, 5 received 8-10 mg/kg/day and 2 received 10-12 mg/kg/day.

In addition to CyA, prednisone was given at a lower dosage than in conventional treatment (7 mg/m^2 at 6 months) and a low dose of AZA (0.7 to 1.5 mg/kg according to GFR). It was planned to stop prednisone after 6 to 8 months of CyA, if renal biopsy allowed it; this phase of the protocol was not yet attained at the time of this report.

II - *Ciclosporin level measurement*

CyA plasma level was measured by radio-immuno-assay. Blood was sampled usually 4 hours after the dose ("peak" level) and before the next dose ("trough" level); after separation of red cells, plasma was stored at room temperature before assay. Measurements were repeated twice weekly until correct dosage was reached, then weekly during 1 month, and twice monthly thereafter.

III - *Renal histology*

In patients treated after 01/01/85, a percutaneous renal biopsy was performed systematically after 4 to 8 months of CyA treatment in order to decide about the withdrawal of prednisone. Earlier samples were obtained in case of unexplained elevation of serum creatinine. Some patients treated before 1985 underwent also a renal biopsy after several months of CyA treatment.

RESULTS

A - *"Primary use"*

I - *Initial use* (1 patient)

This patient, who received his 2nd graft at age 16 in January 1984, was first treated by IV CyA (3 mg/kg/day during the first 2 days), but no detectable serum levels could be obtained (probably because of phenobarbital treatment until day −1), then by oral CyA (14 mg/kg/day). The kidney never functioned, rejection was never controlled, and kidney rupture on day 12 led to transplantectomy.

II - *Early conversion to Ciclosporin* (table I)

1 - *Randomized protocol 1985*

Ten of the 12 patients randomly allocated to CyA after the first month, have a follow-up longer than 3 months on CyA (thus, longer than 4 months post-transplantation). Only 6 have a follow-up > 6 months. One girl lost her graft from rejection 4 months after transplantation, after 15-days withdrawal of CyA for suspected nephrotoxicity. In this case, rejection can be clearly related to this erroneous withdrawal of CyA. Three patients were treated for mild or moderate rejection episodes, occuring respectively 2, 8 and 10 months after transplantation, and at a low dosage of prednisone (0.1 to 0.25 mg/kg/day). Reversibility after methylprednisolone bolus was complete in only one case, while in the other 2, some CyA nephrotoxicity could not be excluded. The

TABLE I

RESULTS ON 01/12/85

RANDOMIZED PROTOCOL

	N (FOLLOW-UP >3 MO)	REJECTION EPISODES	FUNCTIONING GRAFT CREATININE		GRAFT LOSS
			<120 μmol/l	130-200 μmol/l	
CICLOSPORIN	10	4	5	4*	1
CONVENTIONAL TREATMENT	10	3	9	/	1

EARLY ELECTIVE CONVERSION

	FOLLOW-UP	REJECTION	FUNCTIONING GRAFT CREATININE		GRAFT LOSS	NEPHROSIS REMISSION
			< 120 μmol/l	120-150 μmol/l		
N = 5	4—24 MONTHS (Mean = 8)	0	3	2	0	1/1

* 1 CASE WITH SEVERE TUBULOPATHY

other 6 patients did not experience any rejection crisis and had stable renal function.

On 01/12/85, creatinie was ⩽ 120 μmol/l in 5 and 130-200 μmol/l in the other 4 (one of them having suffered from a severe tubulopathy with prolonged anuria). Mean creatinine, excluding this case, was 118 μmol/l. In the control group of 10 patients on conventional treatment with a similar follow-up, the results were the same: one child lost his graft at 3 months from irreversible rejection, 2 were treated for mild rejection episodes at 6 months. Creatinine was ⩽ 120 μmol/l in all 9 patients with functioning grafts (mean = 97 μmol/l).

2 - *Patients with elective conversion before 2 months*

All these 5 patients remained without rejection episodes, during the follow-up ranging from 3 months to 2 years (mean= 9 months). Mean creatinine was 106 μmol/l (84 to 130 μmol/l). The patient with recurrent nephrosis went into remission 3 weeks after starting CyA and has remained almost completely protein-free (≮ 0.30 g/24 h) for 6 months.

B - *Secondary use*

Twenty one patients were converted to CyA for steroid—resistant rejection (table II). Nine of them received CyA during the first month for early severe rejection, with good results; with a mean follow-up of 8 months (2 to 18 months), there was only 1 graft loss; at last examination, creatinine was < 150 μmol/l in 6 patients (although subsequent reversible rejection episodes occurred in some of them) and between 150 and 200 μmol/l in the remaining 2. On the other hand, the results are poor in the 12 children converted after 2 months: 7 graft losses, 3 chronic renal failures and only 2 patients with creatinine < 150 μmol/l. But in this group it should be noted that all children but one experienced one or more pre-existing rejection crises and 6 had chronic rejection at time of conversion.

Among the 11 patients converted after 2 months for non-immunological reasons, there was one graft loss; it concerned a girl converted after 2 years for her third rejection, developing 2 months after AZA withdrawal for anemia. The other 10 patients have a functioning kidney, with a mean follow-up of 11 months (3 mo. to 2 years).

C - *Withdrawal of ciclosporin*

CyA was withdrawn in 7 patients, 2 weeks to 8 months after its introduction; 6 of them had a preexisting chronic rejection with creatininemia <200 μmol/l and CyA was withdrawn because of worsening of renal function or hypertension. Six out of these 7 patients lost their graft, within 2 months for 5 of them.

TABLE II

STEROID-RESISTANT REJECTION

TIME OF REJECTION	N	RESULTS ON 01/12/85 FUNCTIONING GRAFT CREATININE (μmol/l) < 150	> 150	GRAFT LOSS
FIRST MONTH	9	6	2	1
AFTER 1st MONTH	12	2	3	7

D - *Effect on growth*

The beneficial effect on growth is difficult to assess, because of the small number of patients treated for more than 6 months. However, in the group of prepubertal boys (n = 6), a catch-up growth was observed in half the children, and the mean standard deviation score (SDS) of the six patients was positive : + 0.45 SD/ year. The results were poorer in pubertal boys (n = 7), with only 1 catch-up growth. The number of girls with sufficient follow-up is too small to come to a conclusion.

E - *Side effects*

1 - *Nephrotoxicity*

Creatinine level increased in most children when they were converted to CyA. The most important increases (> 50 %) seemed usually related to CyA over-dosage, and were more or less completely reversible by decreasing the dosage. However, a severe acute nephrotoxicity (creatinine x 2 or 3) occurred only twice, in the same child when cotrimoxazole was added to CyA (as previously described [2]), and was completely reversible after withdrawal of cotrimoxazole.

In order to assess more precisely the risk of nephrotoxicity, we studied the renal biopsies performed in our patients, excluding those who had been treated for steroid-resistant rejection. Five biopsies were performed between 1 and 3 months after CyA was started, because of an increase of creatinine : 1 revealed acute rejection, 1 was normal, 1 showed only some foci of tubular epithelial degeneration, and 2 showed a mild acellular fibrosis. Four to eighteen months after treatment started, 10 samples were obtained systematically from children with stable renal function (creatinine < 120 μmol/l in 7, between 150 and 200 μmol/l in 3). Five were normal, 4 showed a mild accellular fibrosis, and 1 surprisingly showed lesions of chronic rejection.

In summary, a mild acellular fibrosis was observed in 6 out of 15 samples, whereas 6 others were normal, without any correlation with present renal function, nor with previous history of tubulopathy of acute reversible rejection. Small arteriolar thrombosis with subintimal hyalinosis was observed in only 2 patients with previous history of severe rejection.

2 - *Other side effects:*

Hypertension was present in the majority of children, but in only 19 cases (40%) it seems to have been triggerred or worsened by CyA prescription. It was however responsible for hypertensive encephalopathy with seizures, fortunately reversible, in 3 patients. Hirsutism was a common finding, noticeable in 20 patients, but it was inconvenient for only 3 girls. Gingival hypertrophy was noted in 3 cases. Tremor was observed in 3 patients but disappeared in 2 of them. Several patients suffered from headaches in case of overdosage. The first child treated in 1982 died after an unexplained coma 2 weeks after CyA withdrawal. Hyperkalemia was present in 3 patients. Neither hepatotoxicity nor noteworthy hypomagnesemia were found. No thrombosis, severe infection or lymphoproliferative disorder were observed.

DISCUSSION

Since corticosteroids are considered the main factor responsible for growth retardation in transplanted children and since it has been claimed that CyA allows to decrease or stop corticosteroids, CyA appears to be the treatment of choice in children with renal allografts [3, 4, 5]. On the other hand, using a new drug with potential nephrotoxicity raises some reluctance, and this preliminary report of CyA use in a pediatric unit is an example of a progressive approach, going from selected indications to systematic administration. Any firm conclusion is impossible from this experience, owing to the various indications, and mainly to the short follow-up of patients entering the randomized protocol. Nevertheless, some points deserve mention and discussion.

In our early experience, two grafts were lost from irreversible rejection in patients receiving preventive CyA treatment. In one case, the preceding phenobarbital treatment probably explains the failure to reach an "active" CyA level during the first day; and in the other one, CyA was wrongly stopped after 2 months in view of an increased creatinine. In all other cases receiving preventive CyA treatment, either in the prospective randomized study (n = 11) or because of cytopenia or recurrent nephrosis (n=5), kidneys are functioning and plasma creatinine is only slightly higer than in patients in conventional treatment.

The number of rejection episodes was lower in the control group but not significantly different, and it should be stressed that this latter group had a higher prednisone dosage than the CyA group. CyA seemed also useful in patients with steroid-resistant rejection occuring during the first month after transplantation, since only one out of 9 such patients lost his graft and 6 of the remaining 8 have plasma creatinine in subnormal range. These results are better than those obtained in our unit during the 3 previous years: among 23 early severe rejection crises, 8 grafts were lost (35 %) and 6 patients (26 %) have chronic renal failure.

As could be expected, CyA was unable to improve patients who already had 2 or 3 rejection episodes and were converted late , more than 2 months after transplantation. On the other hand, withdrawal of CyA in such cases, for fear of nephrotoxicity on an already damaged kidney, is a hazardous procdure, leading most often to an accelerated progresssion to end-stage renal failure.

The growth data during CyA treatment cannot be conclusive, but the 6 prepubertal boys with a follow-up longer than 6 months had a SDS = + 0.45 SD/year, much better than the mean SDS on conventional therapy in our prevous series (− 0.04 SD/year) [6]. These data are in agreement with the preliminary reports on growth of transplanted children treated with CyA alone or with low dose prednisone [4, 5].

With regard to the side effects, only hypertension and nephrotoxicity were a real concern. The role of CyA in hypertension is difficult to evaluate, because in the first year of transplantation, the majority of children have high blood pressure, due to several causes [7]. However, in 40 % of patients, hypertension appeared to have been triggerred or worsened by CyA, and in 3 cases it was responsible for a reversible hypertensive encephalopathy.

A relative nephrotoxicity was evidenced, first by the increase of creatinine level in most cases after CyA was started, often correlated with high CyA levels, and second by the slightly higher creatinine levels in CyA patients compared to the control group, in the randomized protocol. However, renal biopsy failed to show a specific pattern of "nephrotoxicity" in patients with recent or chronic elevation of creatinine. The so-called "CyA specific" tubular lesions [8, 9] were never observed, and arteriolar lesions described by some authors [8, 9] were found only in patients with previous severe rejection crises. Should the slight degree of acellular fibrosis observed in 40% of our patients, and the mild tubular lesions seen in one case, be attributed to CyA toxicity? [10, 11]. In any case, the long-term evlution of these grafts with fibrosis remains a source of concern.

In conclusion, from this short experience, it appears that CyA may bring an improvement in the prognosis of early steriod-resistant rejection, and that, in "primary use", it gives, at least, as good results as the conventional treatment, with probably a beneficial effect on growth.

REFERENCES

1 Hourmant M., Soulillou J.P., Guenel J. Comparison of 3 immunosuppressive strategies in kidney transplantation: antithymocyte globulin and conventional treatment, antithymocyte globulin and Cyclosporin, and Cyclosporin. A one-center randomized study. Transpl Proc 1985; 17:1158–1161.

2 Nyberg G., Gäbel H., Althoff P., Björk S., Herlitz H., Brynger H. Adverse effect of trimethoprim on kidney function in renal transplant patients. Lancet 1984; i:394–395.

3 Conley S.B., Flechner S.M., Gilbert R., Van Buren C.T., Brewer E.D., Kahan B.D. Use of Cyclosporine in pediatric renal transplant recipients J Ped 1985;106:45–49.

4 Klare B., Von Walter J., Hahn H., Emmrich P., Land W. Cyclosporin in renal transplantation in children. Lancet 1984; ii:692.

5 Knight J.F., Roy L.P., Sheil A.G.R. Catch-up growth in children with successful renal transplants immunosuppressed with cyclosporin alone. Lancet 1985; i:159–160.

6 Broyer M., Gagnadoux M-F., Guest G., Busson M.N., Beurton D. Résultats de 310 transplantations de rein de cadavre chez l'enfant et l'adolescent. Arch. Fr. Pediat. 1985; 42:237–243.

7 Broyer M., Guest G., Gagnadoux M-F., Beurton D. Hypertension following renal transplantation in children, Pediatric Nephrology 1987; 1:16-21.

8 Bergstrand A., Bohman S.O., Farnsworth A., Gokel J.M., Krause P.H., Lang W., Mihatsch M.J., Oppedal B., Sell S., Sibley R.K., Thiru S., Verani R., Wallace A.C., Zollinger H.U., Ryffel B., Thiel G., Wonigeit K. Renal histopathology in kidney transplant recipients immunosuppressed with Cyclosporin A: results of an international workshop. Clin. Nephrol. 1985; 24:107–119.

9 Mihatsch M.J., Thiel G., Basler V., Ryffel B., Landmann J., Von Overbeck J., Zollinger H.U. Morphological patterns in Cyclosporin-treated transplant recipients. Transpl. Proc. 1985; 17 (suppl. 1):101–116.

10 Farnsworth A., Hall B.M., Ng. A.B.P., Duggin G.G., Horvath J.S., Sheil A.G.R., Tiller D.J. Renal biopsy morphology in renal transplantation. Am. J. Surg. Pathol. 1984; 8:243–252.

11 Klintmalm G., Bohman S.O., Sudelin B., Wilczek H. Interstitial fibrosis in renal allografts after 12 to 46 months of Cyclosporin treatment: Beneficial effect of low doses in early post transplantation period. Lancet 1984; ii:950–953.

GROWTH, HEALTH AND DEVELOPMENT IN RENAL TRANSPLANTATION IN CHILDREN USING CICLOSPORIN AS PRIMARY IMMUNOSUPPRESSANT

A. TEJANI, K.M.H. BUTT, J. HONG, M.R. KHAWAR, K.D. PHADKE, A. POMRANTZ and M. FUSI

Renal Division, Department of Pediatrics, and the Transplant Service of the Department of Surgery, State University of New York, Health Science Center at Brooklyn, 450 Clarkson Avenue, Box 49, Brooklyn, New York 11203, U.S.A.

Our study shows that 1) children tolerate CyA well with little side effects; 2) it is possible to use CyA as a sole maintenance immunosuppressive in selected recipients of live related and cadaveric organs; 3) CyA can be used as a sole maintenance immunosuppressive in selected patients who start with it at the time of transplant as well as those who are converted from conventional therapy later on, provided they have a stable graft function; 4) all children who have their prednisone withdrawn exhibit adequate endogenous cortisol reserve and 5) the majority of prepubertal children who have discontinued prednisone have sufficient growth hormone reserve to provide a potential for growth.

With improved graft survival, renal transplantation has become the preferred mode of replacement therapy for children in the United States [1]. Despite strides in the post-transplantation rehabilitation of children, the twin problems of growth failure and cushingoid features continue to plague the end results [2]. Both growth failure and the asthetic disfiguration are a direct result of maintenance steroid therapy. Attempts to ameliorate these problems by using alternate day steroid therapy in the conventional regimen has lead to graft rejection in many centers [3].

Rejection in a non-immunosuppressant patient is triggered by an antigen stimulating the macrophage to release Interleukin 1. The mode of action of corticosteroids is by blocking Interleukin 1 production. Ciclosporin (CyA), a peptide fungal derivative appears to have a steroid sparing effect. On a molecular level the drug selectively inhibits the production and/or release of Interleukin 2 from activated T helper cells, which is essential for the proliferation of T lymphocytes [4] and it reduces the release if Interleukin 1 from the macrophages, which is essential for helper cell activation and Interleukin 2 release [5].

CyA has been used at our institution since 1982, for renal transplantation, with the specific aim of utilizing its steroid sparing effect to maintain the renal graft

Correspondence to: A. Tejani, Renal Division, Department of Pediatrics, State University of New York, Health Science Center at Brooklyn, 450 Clarkson Avenue, Box 49, Brooklyn, New York 11203, U.S.A.

on CyA as the sole immunosuppressant. In order to put the efficacy and the toxicity of the drug in children in a proper perspective, this study is limited to children who have received the drug for at least six months or have died prior to the expiration of the six month period. Data is compiled till December 1985.

MATERIALS AND METHODS

Two groups of children were treated with CyA. Group A consisted of 23 children who started with CyA at the time of transplant. 14 children who had received a transplant some time previously, were on conventional therapy – azathioprine (AZA) and prednisone – and were converted from AZA to CyA, form Group B.

The dose of CyA used in patients in Group A was 3 mg/kg intravenously for the first two days, followed by an oral dose of 10 mg/kg beginning day three. The CyA dose was gradually reduced after the first week to achieve a maintenance dose of 6 mg/kg by the 12th week. The post transplant CyA dose was adjusted by weekly whole blood trough level measurements using a high pressure liquid chromatography technique (HPLC). The effective blood level aimed for was between 100–200 ngm/ml.

The prednisone dose used in patients of Group A, was 0.5 mg/kg on the day of transplant This was gradually reduced to 0.1–0.2 mg/kg by 12 weeks. If the renal graft function remained stable, then attempts were made to discontinue prednisone over the next 4–8 weeks.

In patients belonging to Group B, the dose of CyA used was 6 mg/kg oral on the first day of conversion together with ½ the dose of AZA that the patient had been on. On the second day of conversion AZA was discontinued. The CyA dose was adjusted after the first week to obtain a through HPLC between 100–200 ng/ml as in patients of Group A.

The prednisone dose in Group B patients was maintained at the same level as prior to conversion for the first four weeks. If graft function remained stable, attempts were then made to discontinue prednisone over the next 4–8 weeks.

Since there was no previous experience or information available regarding the conversion from AZA to CyA in children, initially patients in Group B were admitted to the hospital for three days to carry out the conversion. As experience was gained, subsequent conversions were carried out in an out-patient setting. As out-patients, children in both groups were monitored weekly or biweekly for evidence of renal dysfunction and CyA hepatotoxicity as needed. Acute rejection episodes in both groups were diagnosed by using the following criteria. 1) Rise in serum creatinine greater than 0.3 mg/dl; 2) evidence of sulphurcolloid uptake on a radionuclide scan [6] and 3) histological evidence of a diffuse lymphocytic infilterate on transplant biopsy. Therapy of rejection consisted of pulse methylprednisolone given in doses of 50–200 mg/day depending upon the weight of the patient for 5–7 days. In some cases where rejection was not reversed by methylprednisolone therapy, antithymocyte globulin was used for 10–14 days. In some cases OKT 3 monoclonal antibody was used to reverse the rejection not responding to other therapy.

Endogenous cortisol measurements

In patients frc both groups who were able to discontinue prednisone, 500 to a 1000 mg of daily NaCl tablets were prescribed from the day of discontinuation for two weeks. At the end of two weeks an ACTH stimulation test was done. A synthetic ACTH (Cortrosyn) was used in the dose of 0.125 mg I.M. for children under two years of age and 0.250 mg I.M. for children older than two years. Blood was drawn for serum cortisol measurement prior to ACTH stimulation and one hour later. If the results of ACTH stimulation revealed adequate endogenous cortisol production, then administration of NaCl tablets was discontinued.

Growth hormone levels

In prepubertal children who were able to discontinue prednisone, growth hormone levels were measured using methyldopa stimulation. Patients were kept fasting overnight, and 500 mg methyldopa was administered per oral. Blood samples were then taken for growth hormone measurements at 0, 20, 40, 60 and 90 and 120 minutes post administration of methyldopa. In some patients growth hormone measurements were carried out on two separate occasions – while still receiving prednisone and a week after discontinuation – in order to determine the influence of prednisone on growth hormone levels.

Statistics

The effect of treatment on survival of patients and grafts was analyzed with the use of product limit estimators of survival curves [7]. Patient and graft survival were calculated separately for both groups. The day of conversion in patients of Group B was considered as the first day of patient and graft survival.

RESULTS

Table 1 shows patient characteristics of Group A, and Table II details factors necessitating conversion in Group B patients.

Patient survival

Fig. 1 shows patient survival in both groups. For patients converted to CyA from conventional therapy, no patient loss has occurred, and actuarial patient survival at 30 months is 100%. 2 patients have died in Group A resulting in 30

TABLE I

Group A (n =23)

Age – range 6 months to 18 years	
Cadaveric Transplant	11
Live Related Transplant	12
First Transplant	14
2nd or 3rd Transplant	9

TABLE II

Group B (n = 14)

Reasons for conversion to Ciclosporin therapy		
1.	Patients with unstable graft	4
2.	Possible growth	5
3.	Steroid toxicity (obesity,acne)	3
4.	Poor compliance on prednisone	2

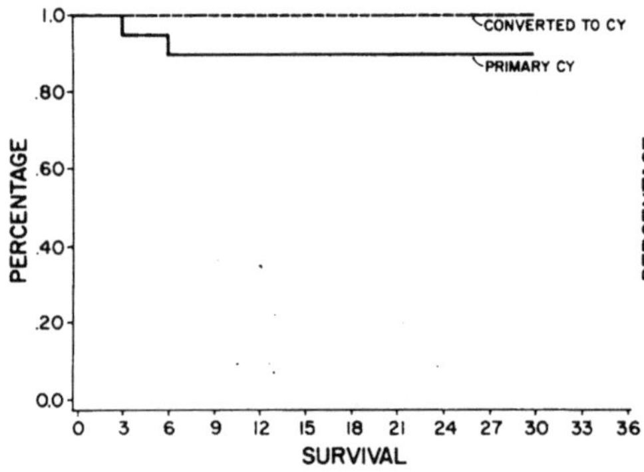

Fig. 1. Patient survival.

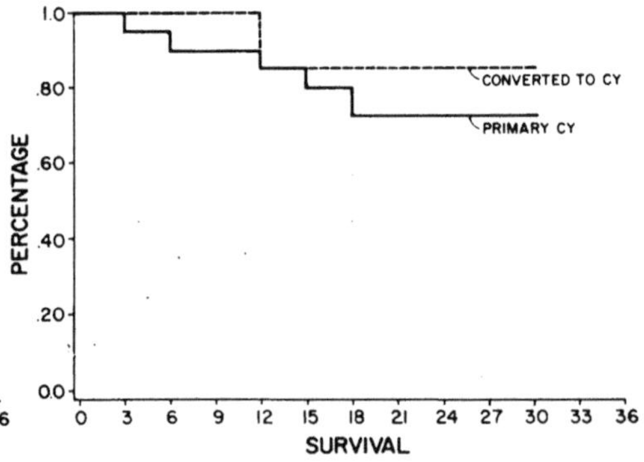

Fig. 2. Graft survival.

months actuarial patient survival of 94%. Both patients were recipients of a 2nd transplant. The first of these patients was an eight year old male with focal segmental sclerosis as the primary disease. He received a live related donor kidney from his father. Five months post transplantation and a month after discontinuing steroid therapy his serum creatinine was 0.6 mg/dl and he was receiving 6 mg/kg of CyA per day. He developed pyrexia 5 months after transplantation and after two days delay he was hospitalized. He died 18 hours after hospitalization of Staphylococcus epidermidis septicemia. The second patient was a 16 years old female recipient of a second cadaveric graft. The graft functioned poorly with an acute rejection episode in the first month and the patient was treated with methylprednisolone for reversal of rejection, following which she developed Herpes viremia and died suddenly. Fig. 2 shows graft survival in both groups. For Group A (primary CyA) 30 month actuarial graft survival is 72% and for Group B (converted to CyA) 30 month actuarial survival is 84%. Graft losses in Group A were all in recipients of a 2nd transplant, where as of the 2 grafts lost in Group B, one was due to noncompliance in a 17 year old female, and the other loss occurring due to chronic rejection in an unstable graft.

Rejection episodes

We calculated the number of rejection episodes in patients in Group B over an 18 month period after converting to CyA therapy and compared them to the episodes of rejection seen in the same group over the previous 18 months, prior to conversion. The mean number of rejection episodes for patient as well as the mean number of days spent in hospital were significantly reduced after conversion. The mean number of rejection episodes per patient were 3.5 (1–10) prior and 1 (0–4) post conversion. The mean number of days in hospital 39 (2–82) was reduced to 10 (0–42) $p<.05$.

Side effects of Ciclosporin therapy

The major side effect of CyA has always been nephrotoxicity. We have considered a rise in serum creatinine greater than 25% over the base line value with a negative sulphur colloid scan and the absence of a lymphocytic infiltration on transplant biopsy as indicative of nephrotoxicity, particularly when associated with a high blood CyA level. Several patients required lowering of the dose but for the duration of this study no patient manifested irreversible nephrotoxicity or necessitated withdrawal of CyA altogether.

TABLE III

Side effects of ciclosporin therapy		
1.	Gingival hyperplasia	11/37
2.	Hypertrichosis	9/37
3.	Seizures	2/37
4.	Anemia	2/37

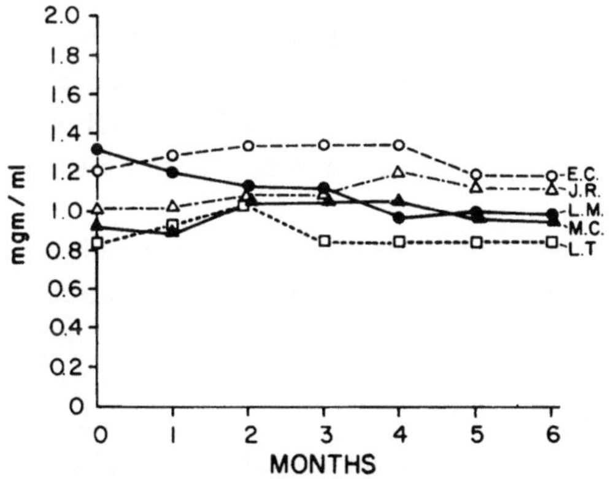

Fig. 3. Serum creatinine during the first six months after discontinuation of prednisone.

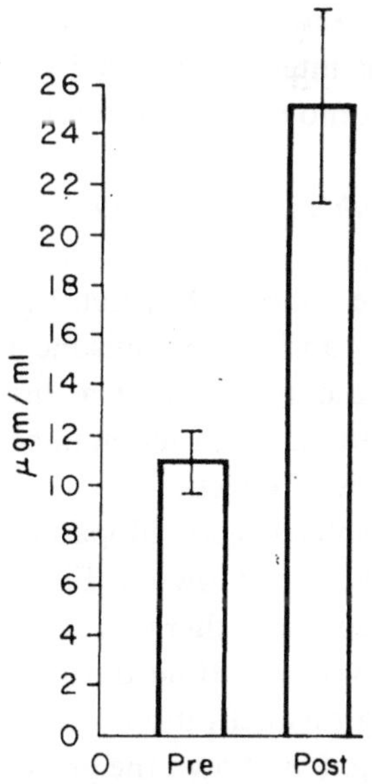

Fig. 4. Serum cortisol pre and post ACTH stimulation.

Other side effects of CyA therapy are shown in Table III. Gingival hyperplasia is seen more frequently in children with poor dental hygiene. Hypertrichosis, where excessive hair growth occurs in a normal distribution, is more frequently observed in children with a darker complexion. This is a concern in adolescent females. Seizures, though seen in only a small percentage of patients, are a major concern since anticonvulsant therapy leads to difficulty in maintaining adequate CyA levels.

Discontinuation of prednisone

A total of 21 children were able to discontinue prednisone, but the drug had to be reinstituted in 7 children because of a rejection episode occurring within 1–3 months. 14 patients have been able to discontinue prednisone from 4–27 months. Eleven of the 14 children belong to Group A, and 3 to Group B. The mean serum creatinine in these 14 patients is 1.1 mg/dl with a range of 0.6 to 1.8 mg/dl.
Fig. 3 shows the serial serum creatinine values of some of the patients plotted over a six month period, after discontinuation of prednisone. Though a transient rise is seen in some of the patients, the serum creatinine at 6 months after discontinuation is unaltered from base line.

Endogenous cortisol production

Fig. 4 shows the mean ± 1 S.D. levels of pre and post ACTH stimulation serum cortisol level in all patients who were able to discontinue prednisone. A two fold rise in serum cortisol following ACTH stimulation shows that the pituitary adrenal axis is intact. Individual values (not shown) revealed all patients to have adequate endogenous cortisol reserve.

Growth and psychological well being

The contrast between the physical features of children on low dose – 5 mg per day – and no prednisone therapy are illustrated in Fig. 5. Fig. 6 shows a 15 year old recipient of a 2nd cadaveric graft with a serum creatinine of 1.1 mg/dl who has been maintained on CyA alone for the last 27 months without a single episode of rejection.

Results of methyldopa stimulated growth hormone levels in some of the prepubertal children are shown in Fig. 7. All five children were examined after discontinuation of prednisone therapy. A stimulated level greater than 10 ng/ml of growth hormone observed any time during the two hour test period is considered to be normal. Using this definition 4 of the 5 children showed adequate growth hormone levels. In Fig. 8 is shown the growth hormone response of another prepubertal child both, while on prednisone therapy, and two weeks after discontinuation of prednisone.

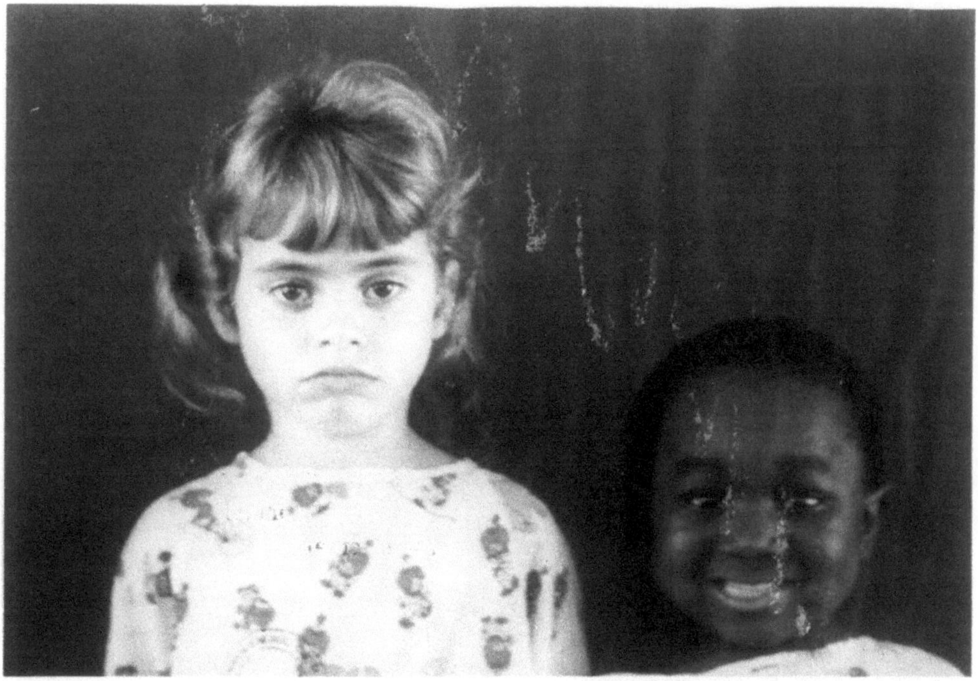

Fig. 5. Two children 6 months post transplant. The girl on the left is not receiving any prednisone, but the boy is on 5 mg/day of prednisone and shows the cushingoid effect.

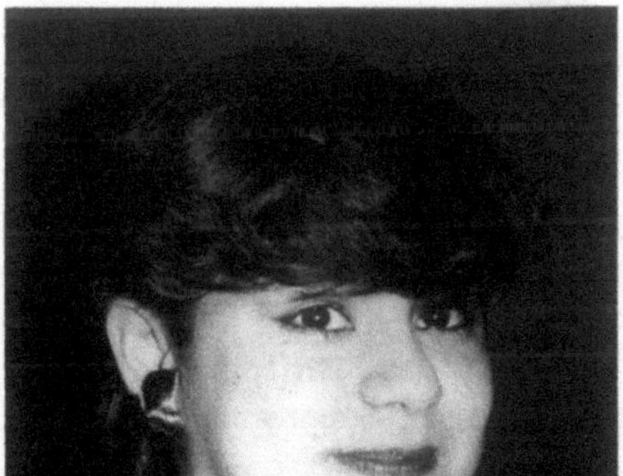

Fig. 6. A 15 year old recipient of a 2nd cadaveric graft, maintained on ciclosporin for 27 months without a single episode of rejection.

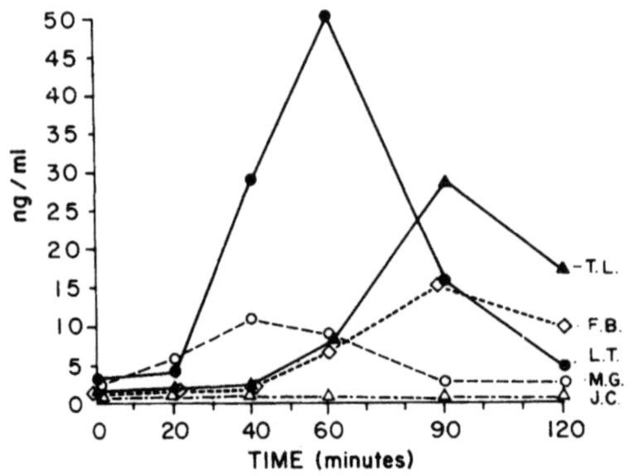

Fig. 7. Growth hormone response to L-DOPA stimulation.

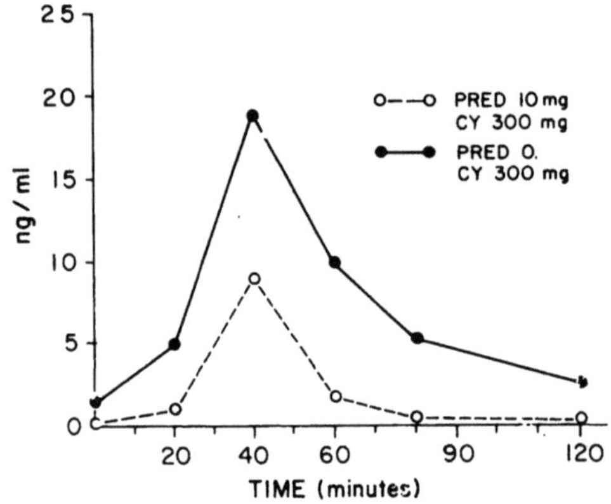

Fig. 8. Growth hormone response to L-DOPA stimulation.

The peak level seen while still under steroid therapy was 9 ng/ml but a peak level of 19 ng/ml was observed after discontinuation.

Fig. 9 and 10 show catch-up growth in boys and girls following discontinuation of prednisone, whereas Fig. 11 shows the remarkable growth spurt in 2 infant boys who are being maintained on CyA as the sole immunosuppressant.

Need for additional prednisone during stress

Fig. 12 shows the serum creatinine values of a 17 year old female who became pregnant one month after discontinuing prednisone. She was the recipient of a second cadaveric transplant, and had a serum creatinine of 1 mg/dl at the time of conception. With the increase in renal blood flow due to the hemodynamics of early pregnancy, she had a decrease in serum creatinine at first. The creatinine stabilized over the next few months and she did not require any additional prednisone throughout her pregnancy.

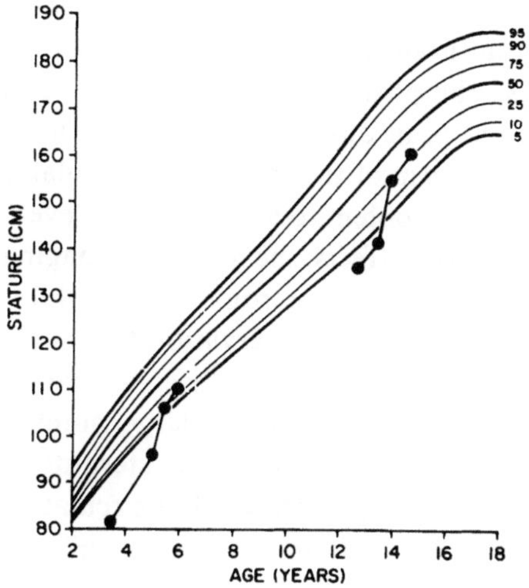

Fig. 9. Growth on ciclosporin (boys).

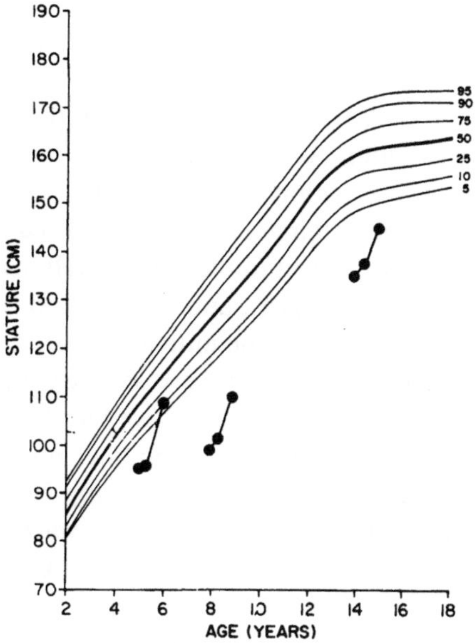

Fig. 10. Growth on ciclosporin (girls).

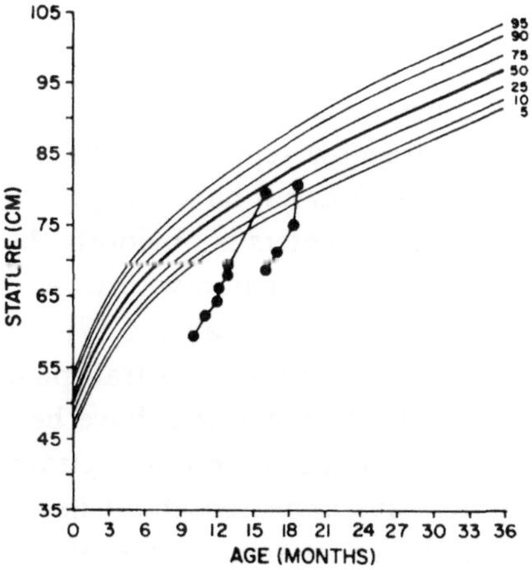

Fig. 11. Growth on ciclosporin (infant boys).

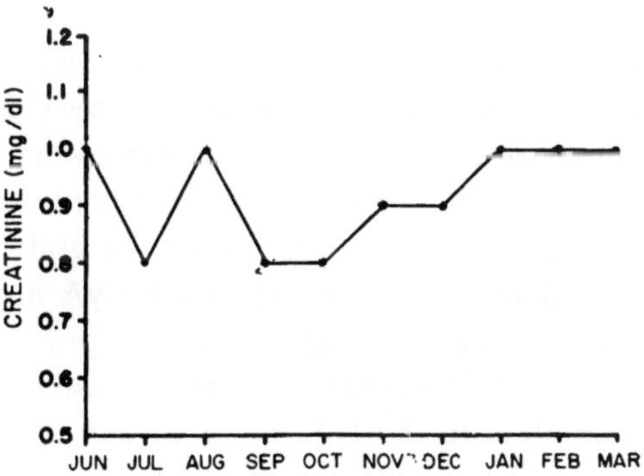

Fig. 12. Serum creatinine through 9 months of pregnancy. Ciclosporin 5 mg/kg.

DISCUSSION

The multiply of side effects seen in patients on maintenance corticosteroids, makes their replacement by a safer more effective chemical immunosuppressive highly desirable. The cushingoid features in transplant patients are subject to individual variations, but are more frequently seen in females, and are probably related to a decreased total body clearance of prednisolone [8]. Non compliance for steroids, due to its esthetic disfigurement is common in young adolescents leading to graft jeopardy [9]. A general consensus among transplant clinicians seems to be that low dose or alternate day therapy with steroids does not alter the facial features of a child. As shown in Fig. 5 this is not an accurate observation, and only the total discontinuation of prednisone can reverse the physiognomy to normal. The relief of cushingoid facies as shown in Fig. 5 and 6, in our study appears to have a salutory effect in the overall well being and self esteem of the children, particularly in adolescent girls, and has reduced the compliance problem to an acceptable level.

In contrast to the individual variation of cushingoid effects, the growth damaging effects of prednisone are seen universally in children. How steroids act to inhibit growth in children is not well understood. In this regard our observation that some of the prepubertal children have higher growth hormone levels after discontinuation of steroid therapy is interesting but needs further confirmation. A large number of theories have been put forward regarding the mode of action of steroids in inducing growth inhibition [10] but the most recent data [11] shows that circulating somatomedin bio-activity fails six hours after steroid administration in children receiving steroid therapy for renal transplant. This would suggest that the normally present somatomedin inhibitors are increased after steroid administration.

Since the majority of prepubertal children in our study showed adequate growth hormone levels, growth potential obviously exists, and the removal of steroid inhibition should provide a growth spurt. In this regard our preliminary data shown in Fig. 9, 10 and 11 are very encouraging. Even other pediatric renal transplant centers who continue to use CyA with prednisone, are now reporting improved height stature in CyA treated patients [12,13,14,15]. CyA does not have any growth stimulating action, hence the improvement noted by other centers is obviously due to the lower maintenance dose of prednisone employed in conjunction with CyA.

The significant improvement in graft survival noted by American [16,17] and Canadian studies [18] has made CyA now an acceptable drug for renal transplantation. However, only scattered reports of the use of CyA in children have been presented. Starzl first reported its use in three children for cadaveric renal retransplantation in the U.S. in 1982 [19], and two reports have appeared about its use in Europe [12,20]. Recently Conley et al [21] have shown its remarkable efficacy (100% patient survival and 83% graft survival) with a mean follow up of 16 months in children.

In the above mentioned studies in children, the drug has been used in conjunction with prednisone. It is not known whether maintenance prednisone is required in patients receiving CyA for renal transplantation [18]. In the European multicenter study [22] 82% of the patients in the CyA group did not receive maintenance prednisone and 27% of the patients never received any steroids. Recent long term evaluation from Cambridge [23] shows that CyA without steroids is capable of sustaining a high percentage of cadaveric renal grafts over a period of 4 years.

Additionally 41% of the CyA treated group in the Cambridge study did not need any steroids. Neither of these studies were controlled, but randomized data from the Canadian [24] study has shown an 84% one year graft survival in patients receiving CyA with steroids, compared to 88% one year graft survival in patients on CyA alone. Unfortunately these groundbreaking studies of using a single maintenance immunosuppressive [22,23,24] were all done on adult patients. Children however have been enrolled in a controlled clinical trial recently done in England, where preliminary results are very encouraging [25].

Our current data support previous observations made in adult graft recipients that serum creatinine levels are higher in patients treated with CyA then in those receiving conventional therapy [26,27]. However, there does not appear to be any further rise in serum creatinine levels after discontinuing prednisone as observed in Fig. 3. Whether the slightly higher serum creatinine levels seen in children with CyA portend a progressive renal functional deterioration is too early to determine, however we have not noted any further rise in serum creatinine levels of children who have stable graft function for 24 months post transplant. Furthermore the most recent data from the Cambridge study shows that stable serum creatinine levels are seen at more than 36 months follow up [23].

Despite a host of techniques used by us and others [6,28,29,30] it is difficult to differentiate nephrotoxicity from rejection. From a controlled trial of high dose CyA vs low dose CyA therapy [31] in our adult transplant recipients, it appears that the incidence of nephrotoxicity is dose related. 66% episodes of renal dysfunction were noted in 64 high dose recipients compared to 14% episodes in 58 low dose recipients ($p<.01$). Our protocol using some of the lowest CyA doses in children ever described, is thus designed to minimize nephrotoxicity. A fall in the level of serum creatinine with a reduction in the dose of CyA particularly when accompanied by an appropriate blood level of CyA appears to be the best retrospective evidence of nephrotoxicity.

Apart from the nephrotoxicity, the only major side effect which merits mention in children is convulsions. 2 of our small children under 6 years of age exhibited seizures while being treated with pulse methylprednisolone during a rejection episode, and needed anticonvulsant therapy. Both phenobarbital and dilantin are known inducers of cytochrome P-450 enzyme system in the liver, causing rapid elimination of CyA from the body. This results in an inability to maintain adequate CyA level for graft tolerance. Higher dose CyA therapy (8–10 mg/kg) divided into 2 or 3 oral doses is necessary in the presence of anti-convulsant therapy.

In the animal model, in the well tolerated dose range (rats up to 17 mg/kg/day and rabbits up to 30 mg/kg/day), CyA has been shown to be without any teratogenic effect [32]. About half a dozen successful pregnancies have been recorded in mothers on CyA without any teratogenicity [33], but most of the babies have been small for gestational age [34,35]. The successful pregnancy in one of our adolescent girls with a baby normal for gestational age would suggest that addition of steroids may have a potential role in producing a small for gestational age baby. Careful monitoring of CyA level and a close watch on the pregnancy appear to be the only additional precautions necessary in patients with good graft function.

REFERENCES

1 Personal communication – Steven Alexander. North American Pediatric ESRD Cooperative Study.
2 Fine R.N., Fine S.E., Malekzadeh M.H. Growth in children following long-term live-related donor allograft: Comparison with long-term cadaver donor allograft function. Symposia Foundation No. 10, Transplantation and Clinical Immunology XVI, Excerpta Medica, 1985.
3 Feldhoff C., Goldman A.I., Najarian J.S., Mauer S.M. A comparison of alternative day and daily steroid therapy in children following renal transplantation. Int. J. Ped. Nephrol. 1984; 5:11–14.
4 Bunjes D., Hardt C., Rollinghof M., Wagner H. Cyclosporin A mediates immunosuppression of primary cytotoxic T cell responses by impairing the releas of interleukin 1 and interleukin 2. Eur. J. Immunol. 1981; 11:657–661.
5 Larsson E.L. Cyclosporin A and dexamethasone suppress T cell responses by selectively acting at distinct sites of the triggering process. J. Immunol. 1980; 124:2828–2833.
6 Trachtmann H., Khawar R., Phadke K., Tejani A. The utility of transplant biopsy, Tc^{99m} sulphur-colloid scan and Cyclosporine drug levels in distinguishing acute rejection versus Cyclosporin nephrotoxicity. Ped. Res. 1985; 19:385A.
7 BMDP Statistical Software PIL Survival Analysis. Univ. of California Press 1983; p 569.
8 Bergrem H., Jervell J., Flatmark A. Prednisolone pharmacokinetics in Cushinoid and non-Cushinoid Lidney transplant patients. Kidney Int. 1985; 27:459–464.
9 Korsch B.M., Fine R.N., Gruskin C.H., Negrete V.E. Experiences with children and their families during extended hemodialysis and kidney transplantation. Ped. Clin. N. Amer. 1971; 18:625–627.
10 Travis L.B., Chesney R., McEnery P, Moel D., Pennisi A., Potter D., Talwalker Y.B., Wolff E.D. Growth and glucocort coids in children with kidney disease. Kidney Int. 1978; 14:365–368.
11 Unterman T., Phillips L.S., Fuso A.C., Mathesan C.K. Steroid induced somatomedin inhibitors. Proc. 65th Annual Meeting American Endocrine Society 1983; p 69.
12 Klare B., Von Walter J., Hahn H., Emmrich P., Land W. Cyclosporin in renal transplantation in children. Lancet 1984; ii:692.
13 Conley S.B. Cyclesporine A serum levels in children. Presented at the 3rd Int. Workshop on Renal insufficiency in Children.
14 Brodehl J. Personal communication.
15 Brewer E.D., Siegler R.L., Alexander D.P., Nelson E.W., Maxwell G.J. Rapid growth in young children after renal transplantation using Cyclosporine and prednisone. Ped. Res. 1985; 19:373A.
16 Starzl T.E., Weil R.I.I.I., Iwatsuki S. The use of Cyclosporine A and prednisone in cadaver kidney transplantation. Surg. Gyn. Obst. 1980; 151:17–26.
17 Kahan B.D., Van Buren C.T., Flechner S.M., Payne W.D., Boileau M., Kerman R.H. Cyclosporine immunosuppression mitigates immunologic risk factors in renal allotransplantation. Transpl. Proc. 1983; 15:2469–2478.
18 The Canadian Multicentre Transplant Study Group. A randomized clinical trial of Cyclosporine in cadaveric renal transplantation. N. Engl. J. Med. 1983; 309:809–815.
19 Starzl T.E., Iwatsuki S., Malatack J.J., Zitelli B.J., Gartner J.C., Hakala T.R., Rosenthal J.T., Shaw B.W. Liver and kidney transplantation in children receiving Cyclosporin A and steroids. J. Ped. 1982; 100:681–686.

20 Hoyer P.F., Offner G., Wonigeit K., Brodehl J., Pichelmayr R. Dosage of Cyclosporine A in children with renal transplants. Cin. Nephrol. 1984; 22:68–71.

21 Conley S.B., Flechner S.M., Gilbert R., Van Buren C.T., Brewer E.D., Kahan B.D. Use of Cyclosporine in pediatric renal transplant recipients J. Ped. 1985; 106:45–49.

22 European Multicenter Trial. Cyclosporine as sole immunosuppressive agent in recipients of kidney allografts from cadaver donors. Lancet 1982; i:57–60.

23 Merion R.M., White D.J.G., Thiru S., Evans D.B., Calne R.Y. Cyclosporine: 5 years experience in cadaveric renal transplantation. N. Engl. J. Med. 1984; 310:148–154.

24 Stiller C. The requirements for maintenance steroids in Cyclosporine-treated renal transplant recipients. Transpl. Proc. 1983; 14:2490–2494.

25 Griffin P.J.A., Gomes Da Costa C.A., Salaman J.R. Renal transplantation without steroids – a controlled clinical trial. Presented at the Int. Symposium on Monitoring and Manipulation in Autoimmune Disease and Organ Transplantation, Montebello, Canada, 1985.

26 Calne R.Y., White D.J.G., Rolles K. Cyclosporine A initially as the only immunosuppressant in 34 recipients of cadaveric organs. Lancet 1979; ii:1033–1036.

27 Hamilton D.V., Calne R.Y., Evans D.B., Thiru S., White D.J.G. The effect of longterm Cyclosporine in renal function. Lancet 1981; i:1218–1219.

28 French M.E., Thompson J.F., Hunnisett A.G.W., Wood R.P M., Morris P.J. Impaired function of renal allografts during treatment with Cyclosporine A nephrotoxicity or rejection. Transpl. Proc. 1983; 15:485–488.

29 Wagner E., Pichelmayr R., Wonigeit K., Klempnauer J., Bunzendahl H., Lauchart W. Differentiation between rejection and Cyclosporin A nephrotoxicity by monitoring interstitial pressure in human renal allografts Transpl. Proc. 1983; 15:489–492.

30 Klintmalm G., Bergstrand A., Ringden O. Graft biopsy for the differentiation between nephrotoxicity and rejection in Cyclosporin A treated renal transplant recipients. Transpl. Proc. 1983; 15:493–496.

31 Hong J., Quinto E., Manis T., Butt K.H.M. Impact of high and low Cyclosporine doses on early renal allograft function. Presented at the 4th Annual Symposium of the North American Society for Dialysis and Transplantation.

32 Data provided by Medical Services Dept. Pharmaceutical Division, Sandoz. Inc.

33 Lewis G.J., Lamat C.A.R., Lee H.A., Slapak M. Successful pregnancy in a renal transplant recipient taking Cy A. Br. Med. J. 1983; 286:603.

34 Klintmalm G., Althoff P., Appleby G., Segerbrandt E. Renal function in a newborn baby delivered of a renal transplant patient taking Cyclosporine. Transplantation 1984; 38:198–199.

35 Flechner S.M., Katz A.R., Rogers A.J., Van Buren C.T., Kahan B.D. The presence of Cyclosporine in body tissues and fluids during pregnancy. Am. J. Kid. Dis. 1985; 1:60–63.

CICLOSPORIN AND PREDNISONE IMMUNOSUPPRESSION IN PEDIATRIC RECIPIENTS OF RENAL ALLOGRAFTS

S.M. FLECHNER, S.B. CONLEY, G. ROSE, C. VAN BUREN, R. KERMAN, M. LORBER and B.D. KAHAN

From the Departments of Surgery and Pediatrics, the Division of Immunology and Organ Transplantation, The University of Texas Medical School at Houston.

CyA and prednisone were used to immunosuppress 34 pediatric renal allograft recipients between the age of 1.5 and 16 years. The group included 17 recipients of living related kidneys and 17 recipients of mismatched cadaveric kidneys. The 4 year graft survival is 82% for recipients of living donor grafts and the 3 1/2 year graft survival is 72% for the cadaveric recipients. There was no mortality during this follow up interval. Hirsutism and hypertension were the most frequently observed side effects of this regimen, but no child required discontinuation of CyA therapy. The incidence of rejection episodes was 38% [13/34]. There was no evidence of chronic deterioriation in renal function up to 4 years. CyA and prednisone are demonstrated to be a relatively safe regimen for children, which permits acceptable renal function and linear growth in the pediatric population.

During the past five years Ciclosporin (CyA) in combination with steroids has been emerging as the preferred immunosuppressive regimen for recipients of human organ allografts. Initial favorable experiences in recipients of cadaveric (CAD) renal allografts [1,2] led to further trials in living related (LRD) renal recipients[3] as well as heart, liver, bone marrow, and pancreas recipients[4]. Most of the above protocols were confined to adult patients. At the University of Texas Medical School at Houston, CyA was introduced in adult patients during the fall of 1980. Our encouraging early experience with CyA in adults lead to its incorporation into the pediatric program in the fall of 1981[5].

The major obstacles to standardized CyA therapy were evident during the initial clinical investigations. They include a drug induced nephrotoxicity, and a varible metabolism which necessitates an individualized approach to administration[6,7]. The use of CyA in children would be severely limited if drug induced nephrotoxicity produced a chronic renal dysfunction which prevented post transplant growth and development. In addition, any advantage in graft survival would be lost if the incidence of treated rejection episodes resulted in a greater cumulative dose of steroids

---

Correspondence to: S.M. Flechner, Stanford University Medical Center, Division of Transplantation S-283, 300 Pasteur Drive, Stanford, California 943305, U.S.A.

for CyA treated children. Our experience during the past four years with CyA and Prednisone in children from 1.5 to 16 years of age is presented herein.

MATERIALS AND METHODS

Patients

The patient population included 34 children who received renal transplants between September, 1981 and September, 1985 at The University of Texas Medical School at Houston. The children were aged 1.5 to 16 (mean 10.5) years at the time of transplantation, and received only CyA and prednisone as immunosuppressive agents. There were 20 males and 14 females, 26 of whom were prepubertal. Seventeen patients received mismatched cadaver kidneys, 10 of which came from pediatric donors under age 10. Seventeen children received haploidentical living related kidneys, 16 of which were from parental and one from a sibling donor. The etiology of ESRD included Glomerulonephritis 9, Dysplasia with Reflux or Obstruction 11, Posterior Urethral Valves 4, Hereditary Nephritis 2, Eagle-Barrett Syndrome 2, Polycystic Disease 2, Renal Hypoplasia 2, Congenital Nephrotic Syndrome 1, and Primary Oxalosis 1.

Pretransplant Preparation

As part of our protocol, no intentional third party or donor specific blood transfusions were given prior to transplantation. However, at least two historical third party units were given to 11 LRD and 12 CAD recipients prior to transplant evaluation. Pretransplant nephrectomies were done in 16 children, and one had received a splenectomy. Seven children underwent primary transplantation, and had never been on chronic dialysis. Twenty were treated by hemodialysis and 7 by peritoneal dialysis prior to transplant. Cadaver recipients were transplanted with an attempt to assign the best tissue type available. However, poor matches were never excluded when a crossmatch negative blood type compatible organ became available. Therefore 6 patients received > 2 HLA A,B matched kidneys and 11 patients < 2 A,B matched kidneys. There were no 2 Dr matches, nine 1 Dr matches, and eight 2 Dr mismatches.

Immunosuppression

Prior to transplantation recipients of CAD kidneys were given 14mg/kg of CyA orally. The LRD recipients usually received I.V. CyA by continuous infusion for five days at a dose of 6 mg/kg per 24 hours for small children ($<$ 20 kg) and 3 mg/kg per 24 hours for larger children. No CyA was given intraoperatively, and the I.V. infusion was restarted post-operatively until ileus was resolved, usually by day 3. The 14 mg/kg oral dose was tapered to 12 mg/kg weeks 2-3; 10 mg/kg weeks 4-12; and thereafter adjusted to keep serum trough levels at 50-100 ng/ml (radioimmunoassay determinations) [8]. Children who demonstrated a short T 1/2 on pharmakokinetic analysis were given B.I.D. or T.I.D. dosing schedules. Steroids were begun intraoperatively with a dose of 125-250 mg methylprednisolone. Post-operatively, prednisone was begun at 2 mg/kg and tapered rapidly to 0.5 mg/kg the first week; 0.25 mg/kg at one month; down to a maintenance dose of 0.10-0.15 mg/kg by three months.

Renal Function

Episodes of renal dysfunction associated with elevated CyA trough levels (> 200 ng/ml) were treated by dose reduction of 25-100 mg/day. Progressive renal dysfunction associated with low CyA levels (< 50 ng/ml) prompted renal biopsy. Rejection episodes were confirmed by renal biopsy when possible. They were treated with I.V. steroids at 15-20 mg/kg followed by recycling oral steroids beginning at 3 mg/kg. Renal function is reported at intervals post-transplant as mg/dl. Twenty-four hour creatinine clearances were measured in children during outpatients visits. Some interval creatinine clearances could not be measured in several small children who remained in diapers.

Growth

The height of each child in centimeters (cm) was recorded prior to transplantation. Linear growth measurements for those children with a functioning graft for at least one year were plotted in standard curves adapted from National Center For Health Statistics, Hyattsville, Maryland publications [9]. Each child exhibited significant weight gain post transplant which was not considered a suitable marker for growth.

RESULTS

Transplant Outcome

For the entire follow up period ranging from 3 to 51 months, there has been no mortality. Figure 1 provides the CAD graft survival which was 87% at one year and 76% at two years. Figure 2 provides LRD graft survival which was 82% out to four years post-transplant.

There were 3 LRD graft losses. In two cases, severe steroid resistent accelerated rejection lead to transplant nephrectomy during the first week post-transplant. A third patient with focal sclerosing glomerulonephritis developed heavy proteinuria (> 15 gm per 24 hours) and recurrent disease during the first few weeks post-

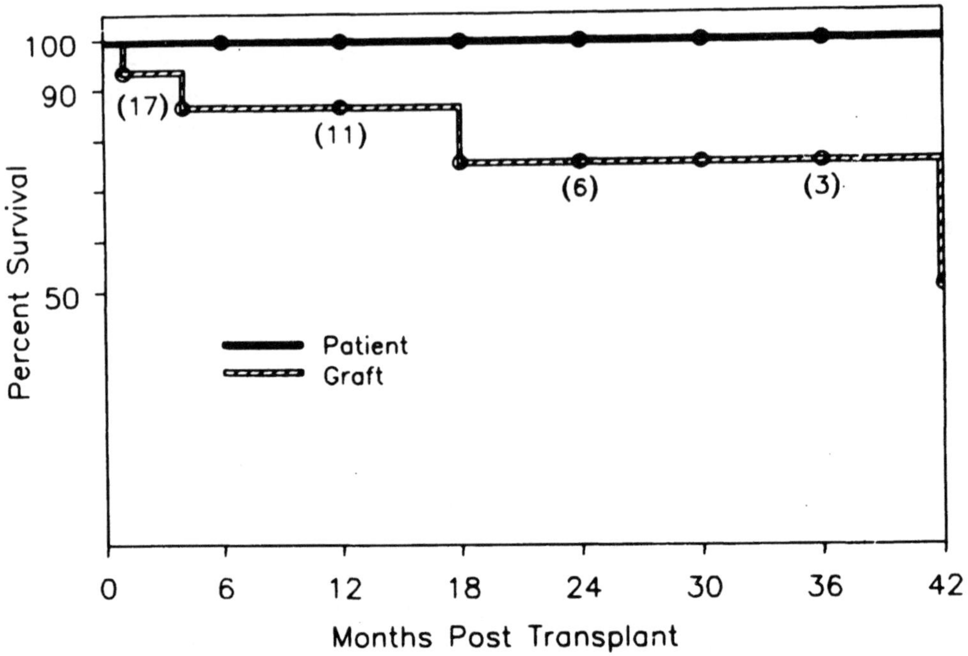

Figure 1. Cadaver graft survival in pediatric recipients using life table methods. Numbers in parentheses represent number of patients at risk.

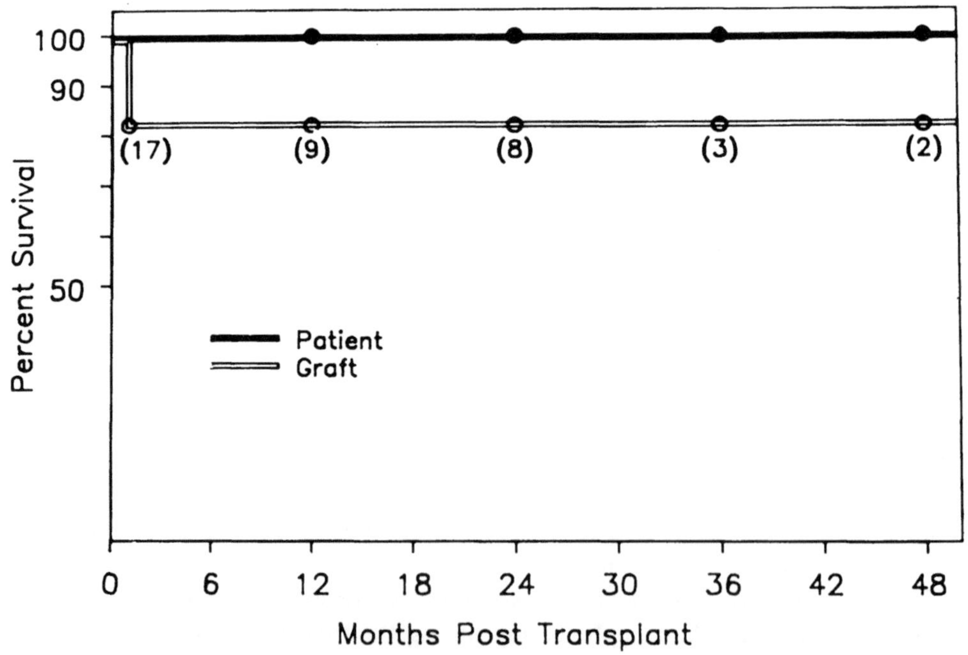

Figure 2. Living related donor graft survival in pediatric recipients using life table methods. Numbers in parentheses represent number of patients at risk.

transplant which eventuated in transplant nephrectomy at one month. There were 4 CAD graft losses including one case of primary nonfunction, probably caused by ongoing rejection. Two grafts were lost to chronic rejection at 14 and 40 months. One child with primary oxalosis developed recurrent oxalate deposition and renal dysfunction leading to graft loss at four months. Interestingly, in the CAD population, 3 of the 4 graft losses occurred in retransplant patients. The overall graft survival for first CAD graft recipients was 10/10 for those at risk for at least one year, and 6/7 for those at risk two years.

Allograft Rejection

In the LRD population only 7/17 [41%] of children experienced a rejection episode, and in the CAD population only 6/17 [35%] required antirejection therapy. Six of the 7 LRD rejection episodes occurred during the first month post-transplant, while the CAD rejection episodes occurred during the first, second, seventh, twelth, and eighteenth months.

Laboratory Values

Tables I and II provide pertinent laboratory values post-transplant for both the CAD and LRD populations, respectively. It is evident that for each population the daily dose of CyA decreased with time, and stabilized at 5-7mg/kg per day after several years. The mean serum CyA trough levels at each interval were higher

TABLE I

Laboratory Values in CAD Recipients Post Transplant (mean ± SE)

months	6	12	18	24	30	36
n	14	12	9	5	5	4
CyA (mg/kg)	7.8 ±.85	7.7 ±.77	6.9 ±.75	6.3 ±.81	5.8 ±.81	5.3 ±.94
CyA trough (ng/ml)	91 ±10	86 ±11	73 ±12	65 ±16	78 ±25	74 ±18
creatinine (mg/dl)	1.12 ±.38	1.21 ±.42	1.31 ±.20	1.51 ±.10	1.50 ±.19	1.47 ±.22
creatinine clearance (ml/min.)	61 ±8.3	62 ±6.8	63 ±6.7	56 ±6.3	58 ±3.6	60 ±2.1

TABLE II

Laboratory Values in LRD Recipients Post Transplant (mean ± SE)

months	6	12	18	24	30	36	42
n	14	11	8	8	6	3	2
CyA (mg/kg)	9.1 ±.73	7.8 ±.91	7.1 ±1.1	6.5 ±1.3	6.5 ±1.3	7.1 ±1.2	5.7 ±2.3
CyA trough (ng/ml)	58 ±11	49 ±10	38 ±8.7	35 ±5.8	33 ±6.7	37 ±8.5	36 ±7.0
Creatinine (mg/dl)	1.01 ±.13	1.14 ±.15	1.30 ±.21	1.13 ±.19	1.24 ±.21	1.60 ±.31	1.40 ±.30
Creatinine clearance (ml/min.)	56 ±3.8	61 ±3.6	58 ±3.8	63 ±8.5	74 ±6.9	63 ±6.9	65 ±6.4

for CAD recipients, even though they were usually receiving slightly less CyA per day. The mean serum creatinine values remained stable for both the CAD and LRD recipients at each interval, with no apparent deterioration with time. This was also observed in the mean creatinine clearance values which remained stable throughout the follow up interval.

Complications

Significant post-transplant infectious complications included 13 bacterial infections, 6 viral infections, and 3 fungal infections. Each required in-patient therapy. One 4-year-old LRD recipient suffered initial ureteral necrosis post-transplant requiring operative repair. Since then he has had 4 severe bouts of pyelonephritis. Three children suffered severe bouts of viral gastroenteritis necessitating intravenous fluid replacement and CyA administration.

Side effects considered to be associated with CyA and prednisone therapy are reported in Table III. Hirsutism was the most frequently encountered side effect in the pediatric population. This was destressing to several female patients, who required applications of depilatory cream. Five children required antiseizure medication post-transplant, two of which had a previous history of seizure disorders. No localizing neurological findings could be identified in the others. Hepatotoxicity defined as transaminase elevations (twice normal) and bilirubin > 2 mg/dl was uncommon and responded to dose reduction. No child had CyA discontinued for an uncontrolled side effect.

TABLE III

SIDE EFFECTS IN PEDIATRIC PATIENTS TREATED WITH CyA AND PREDNISONE IMMUNOSUPPRESSION

N	CAD 17	LRD 17	TOTAL 34
Hepatotoxicity	2	1	3
Hirsutism mild	10	9	19
severe	2	2	4
Tremor	4	5	9
Seizures	2	3	5
Gum Hyperplasia	0	0	0
Hypertension	12	7	19
Osteonecrosis	1	2	3
Tumors	0	0	0

Linear Growth Determinations

Figures 3 and 4 demonstrate the linear growth achieved by those children who had a functioning renal allograft for at least one year. Four female and 7 male recipients of LRD kidneys and 5 female and 6 male recipients of CAD kidneys demonstrated continued linear growth post transplant. Some children experienced growth acceleration and catch up growth. However, many of the older children had curves which continued to be flatter than those predicted for non ESRD children.

DISCUSSION

The preferred management of children with ESRD has been controversial since the availability of maintenance dialysis and clinical renal transplantation. However, renal transplantation has been gaining a wider acceptable during the past decade in many centers in North America and Western Europe. Coincident with this increased activity has been a reappraisal of clinical outcome. Reports of crude survival are no longer adequate, as emphasis has shifted to the return to pre-illness levels of growth and development [10]. In addition, small infants, previously excluded from ESRD care, are entering the pool of potential transplant recipients. Although successful renal transplantation appears to permit the maximal opportunity for growth in these children, allograft rejection and the consequences of its treatment continue to diminish the potential for rehabilitation in many pediatric transplant patients.

CyA, a fungal endecapeptide with distinct lipophilic properties has been introduced as a potent immunosuppressive agent. Widely used in combination with prednisone, the agent appears to suppress the proliferation of allo-reactive T-lymphocytes. It

Growth in Female Pediatric Recipients of CAD Kidneys Treated with Ciclosporin.

Growth in Male Pediatric Recipients of CAD Kidneys Treated with Ciclosporin.

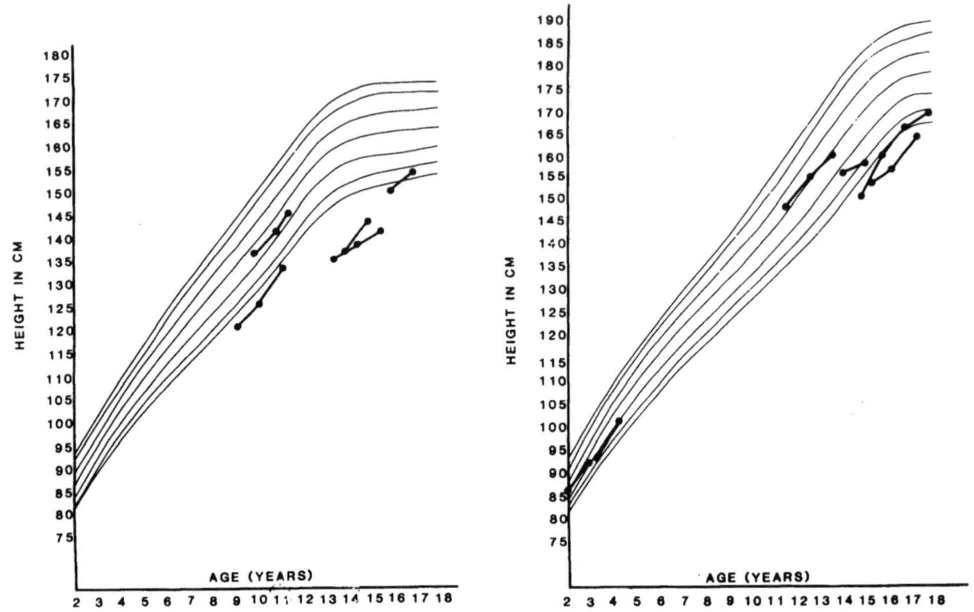

Figure 3. Linear growth of cadaveric recipients after transplant Patients with at least one year of graft function were recorded. Growth charts adapted from National Center for Health Care statistics. Curves represent 5 th, 10th, 25th, 50th, 75th, 80th, and 95th percentiles for age.

has been demonstrated that CyA interrupts the necessary cellular signals for lymphocyte interactions, yet spares the functional capacity of granulocytes, platelets, and red blood cells. A major concern for pediatric patients in that CyA associated nephrotoxicity would lead to chronic renal dysfunction and growth impairment.

This report confirms our previous short term observations that the use of CyA in the pediatric population is associated with improved allograft survival, diminished complications, and acceptable levels of renal function which permit growth and development [11]. These has been no mortality for these children up to 51 months post-transplant. The 4 year LRD graft survival of 82% and the 3 1/2 year CAD graft survival of 72% are essentially the same as we have achieved in adult recipients [12]. In addition, the incidence of rejection episodes (35-40%) and their time of occurrence (usually during the first month post-transplant) also mirror the experience of adult patients.

Nephrotoxicity has not been a serious problem in the pediatric age group, and there has been no apparent trend toward chronic renal deterioration up to 4 years. The mean values for 24 hour creatinine clearances (uncorrected for size) have remained between 50-60 ml/min at each follow up interval. One explanation for this may be that younger patients exhibit a more rapid clearance of CyA with

Growth in Female Pediatric Recipients of LRD Kidneys Treated with Ciclosporin.

Growth in Male Pediatric Recipients of LRD Kidneys Treated with Ciclosporin.

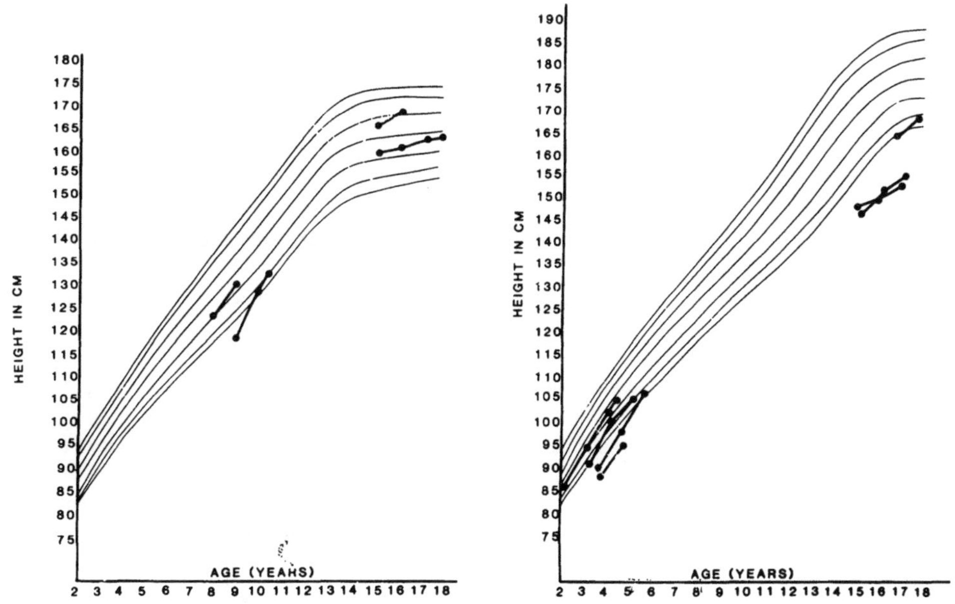

Figure 4. Linear growth of LRD recipients after transplant. Patients with at least one year of graft function were recorded. Growth charts adapted from, National Center for Health Care Statistics. Curvers represent 5th, 10th, 25th, 50th, 75th, 80th, and 95th precentiles for age.

subsequent lower serum trough levels. The importance of pharmakokinetic studies is emphasized in those patients who demonstrate T 1/2 ≤ 8-10 hours. Such patients do well with a divided dose schedule. This approach will also avoid the use of suprapharmacologic doses (> 20 mg/kg) which can predispose to other toxic or infectious complications.

While it is generally agreed that the ultimate adult height achieved by the pediatric ESRD patient will be depressed [13], nearly all CyA treated children demonstrated continued linear growth. It appears however, that only the younger children experience catch up growth and that postpubertal patients have a very flat growth curve.

The experience in pediatric renal transplantation using CyA and prednisone at our center has yielded excellent patient and graft survival with acceptable morbidity. Although tissue typing and prospective blood transfusions did not appear to have major impact on graft survival, it is evident that even with CyA retransplant patients are at high risk for subsequent rejection. This experience has also been observed in our adult population [14]. These data suggest that more attention to tissue typing may be prudent for the patient with a previously failed graft.

In conclusion, CyA and prednisone continue to be a relatively safe and efficacious immunosuppressive regimen for pediatric recipients of both CAD and LRD renal allografts up to 4 years post-transplant. CyA induced nephrotoxicity has not been a serious problem in this population, and no child has required discontinuation of CyA for toxic side effects. The realization of the full growth potential and rehabilitation of these children will await an additional extended period of observation.

REFERENCES

1 European Multicentre Trial Group. Cyclosporin in cadaveric renal transplantation: One year follow-up of a multicentre trial. Lancet 1983; ii:986–989

2 The Canadian Multicentre Transplant Study Group. A randomized clinical trial of Cyclosporine in cadaveric renal transplantation. N. Engl. J. Med. 1983; 309:809–815

3 Flechner S.M., Kerman R.H., Van Buren C.T., Payne W.D, Kahan B.D. The use of Cyclosporin and prednisone for high MLC haploidentical living related transplants. Transpl. Proc. 1983; 15:442–445

4 Kahan B.D., (ed). The first international congress on Cyclosporine. Transpl. Proc. 1983; 15 (suppl 1):2207–3107

5 Conley S.B., Brewer E.D., Flechner S.M., Van Buren C.T., Kahan B.D. Renal transplantation using Cyclosporine in pediatric patients 3 to 17 years old. Transpl. Proc. 1983; 15:2528–2530

6 Flechner S.M., Van Buren C.T., Kerman R.H., Kahan B.D. The nephrotoxicity of Cyclosporine in renal transplant recipients. Transpl. Proc. 1983; 15:2689–2694

7 Kahan B.D., Van Buren C.T., Lin S.N., Yoshinari O., Agostino G., LeGrue S., Boileau M., Payne W.D., Kerman R.H. Immunological monitoring of Cyclosporin A-treated recipients of cadaveric kidney allografts. Transplantation 1982; 34:36–45

8 Donatsch P., Abisch E., Homberger M., Traber R., Trapp M., Voges R. A radioimmunoassy to measure Cyclosporine A in plasma and serum samples. J. Immunoassay 1981; 2:19–32

9 Hamill P.V.V., Drizd T.A., Johnson C.L., Reed R.B., Roche A.F., Moore W.M. Physical growth. National Center for Health Statistics percentiles. Am. J. Clin. Nutr. 1979; 32:607–629

10 Fine R.N. Renal transplantation in children J. Ped. 1982; 100:754–755

11 Flechner S.M., Conley S.B.. Van Buren C.T., Rose G., Kerman R.H., Kahan B.D. Impact of Cyclosporin on renal function and growth in pediatric renal transplant recipients. Transpl. Proc. 1985; 17:1284–1288

12 Kahan B.D., Van Buren C.T., Flechner S.M., Jarowenko M., Yasumura T., Rogers A.J., Yoshimura N., LeGrue S., Drath D., Kerman R.H. Clinical and experimental studies with Cyclosporine in renal transplantation. Surgery 1985; 97:125–140

13 Pennisi A.J., Costin G., Phillips L.S., Malekzadeh M.H. Somatomedin and growth hormone studies. In pediatric renal allograft recipients who receive daily prednisone. Am. J. Dis. Childh. 1979; 133:950–954

14 Flechner S.M., Lorber M.I., Kerman R.H., Van Buren C.T., Wideman C., Kahan B.D. Does Cyclosporine influence the results of cadaver retransplantation? Human Immunol 1985; 14:305–313.

LONG TERM USE OF CICLOSPORIN: SIDE-EFFECTS AND GROWTH FOLLOWING PEDIATRIC KIDNEY TRANSPLANTATION

G. OFFNER, P.F. HOYER, H. JUEPPNER, J. BRODEHL

Department of Pediatric Nephrology, Medical School Hannover, P.O. Box 610180, D-3000 Hannover 61, Federal Republic of Germany.

CyA is a potent immunosuppressive drug which has mainly transient side effects. A main advantage is the normal growth, observed after renal transplantation. However, CyA-induced nephrotoxicity remains a major concern.

PATIENTS AND METHODS

Since September 1982, 50 children (age 2–16 years) who received a kidney transplantation in our center were treated with Ciclosporin (CyA) and low-dose prednisolone (Table 1). Fourty-three patients were treated primarily according to the procotol published by Hoyer et al. [1]. Seven children were converted from conventional immunosuppression with azathioprine (AZA) to CyA which was started with a dose of 250 mg/m²/body surface area. When the trough blood levels of CyA were within the therapeutic range of 250 ng/ml to 500 ng/ml, usually after 3 days, AZA was discontinued and prednisolone reduced to a dose of 4 mg/m²

RESULTS

Out of 50 patients, one child died of Klebsiella sepsis, 3 are back on hemodialysis or CAPD. The remaning 46 children are alive with a functioning graft.

Out of the 43 children primarily treated with CyA, 7 children were switched to a triple therapy, a combination of AZA, CyA and prednisolone. The protocol for triple immunosuppression is summarized in Table II. CyA is reduced to 150 mg/m² body surface area or 5 mg/kg body weight in order to keep CyA blood level between 100–200 ng/ml.

Prednisolone is given in a dose similar to the CyA regimen. AZA is added in dose of 60 mg/m² body surface area or 2 mg/kg body weight. The 7 patients on triple therapy are listed in Table III. The medical indication for triple therapy was a

Correspondence to: G. Offner, Department of Pediatric Nephrology, Medical School Hannover, P.O. Box 610180, D-3000 Hannover 61, Federal Republic of Germany.

TABLE I

Immunuosupression after kidney transplantation with CyA

	N	died	HD/CAPD	Functioning Graft
Primary	43	1	2	40
Conversion from AZA	7	–	1	6
Total	50	1	2	46

TABLE II

Triple immunosuppression

	mg/m²	mg/kg	blood level ng/ml
CyA	150	5	100–200
Prednisolone	4	0.1	
AZA	60	2	

TABLE III

Course after conversion from CyA to triple immunosuppression

Pat	Indication	months P. Tx	CyA dosage mg/m²	blood level ng/ml	Serum creat. pre/post μmol/l	CyA after conversion dosage mg/m²	blood level ng/ml
P H	toxicity	29	150	371	312/236	115	480
S K	chron rej.	23	220	238	311/316	170	143
U B	imp.renal f.	22	220	288	375/HD	-	
B R	imp.renal f.	18	270	412	245/143	160	135
N D	8 acute rej.	18	270	269	400/340	150	172
N K	toxicity	16	250	369	277/190	150	133
A L	4 acute rej.	7	330	449	235/250	250	228

histologically confirmed CyA-toxicity in 2 patients, frequent acute rejection episodes in two children and chronic rejection or impaired renal function in three patients. Triple therapy was initiated 7 months to 29 months post transplantation. CyA dosage at that time ranged between 150–330 mg/m². CyA blood levels were between 238 to 449 ng/ml, thus indicating no evidence for toxic levels. Renal function was reduced in all patients.

After conversion to triple therapy one patient went into endstage renal failure and two patients had no change in serum creatinine levels. In the remaining four patients the kidney function improved as indicated by decrease in serum creatinine of 60–102 μmol/l. CyA blood levels ranged between 133 and 480 ng/ml.

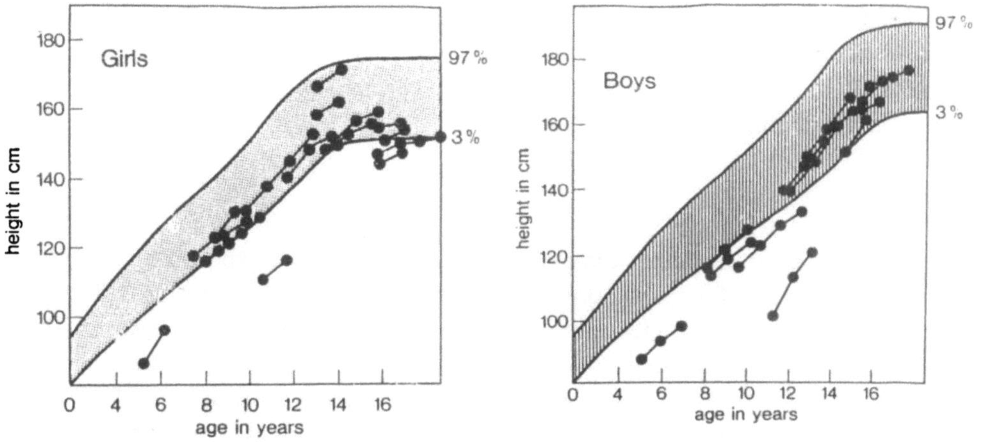

Fig. 1. Indiv'dual growth curves of 13 boys and 16 girls following kidney transplantation with CyA compared to Tanner's reference population.

SIDE EFFECTS

Hypertension occured in 52% of the 50 transplanted patients using CyA. It is the most frequent extrarenal side effect (Table IV). The hypertensive problems in CyA treated patients are less frequent than with conventional therapy (incidence of 80% hypertension). Troublesome hirsutism occured in 36% of the patients. Tremor and paresthesia were dependent on the CyA dosage and va ished with reduction. Six % of the patients developed gingival hyperplasia. Within the first two weeks post transplantation two children presented with seizures, which were at least in 1 patient related to hypomagnesiemia. One child with hyperuricemia suffered from a gout attack, a 16-years old girl

TABLE IV

Extrarenal toxicity of CyA (N=50)

	N	%
Hypertension	31	62
Hirsutism	18	36
Tremor/paresthesia	7	14
Infections	6	12
Gingival hyperplasia	3	6
Convulsion	2	4
Hyperuricemia with gout	1	2
Mammary fibroadenomas	1	2
Localized edema	1	2
Alveolitis	1	2

developed benign mammary fibroadenomas, 1 child developed a Quincke like localized edema, 1 child had a alveolitis. Viral and bacterial infections were observed in 6 cases (12%), cytomegaly in one patient, herpes simplex in 2, osteomyelitis in 1 and septic complications in 2 patients.

GROWTH

A major reason to start with CyA therapy in children was the expectation of a better growth rate because of the lower prednisolone dosage in long term treatment. Twenty-nine transplanted children (13 boys and 16 girls) who had at least one year of graft function, could be evaluated. The individual growth curves are compared to Tanner's reference population. All of them grew normally or showed catch up growth (Fig. 1).

According to the stage of pubertal development, the individual annual growth rates, expressed as standard deviation score (SDS), remained stable or improved after transplantation. Prepubertal boys had the lowest SDS with −3.8, prepubertal girls had −3.0. The pubertal and postmenarchal girls as well as the postpubertal boys revealed a low mean level of SDS, which is still within the normal range (Table V).

TABLE V

Growth after kidney transplantation with CyA

SDS of height	N	at Tx	1.yr	2.yr
Boys	13			
prepub.stage	4	−3.8	−3.6	−3.6
pub.stage	4	−3.1	−2.4	−2.3
postpub.stage	5	−0.9	−0.7	—
Girls	16			
prepub.stage	5	−3.0	−2.7	—
pub.stage	3	−1.7	−1.4	—
postmenarchal	8	−1.8	−1.5	−1.3

REFERENCES

1 Hoyer P.F., Offner G., Wonigeit K., Brodehl J., Pichelmayr R. Dosage of Cyclosporine A in children with renal transplants. Clin Nephrol 1984; 22:68–71.

RENAL FUNCTION IN CHILDREN TREATED WITH CICLOSPORIN AFTER RENAL TRANSPLANTATION. A COMPARISON WITH CONVENTIONAL IMMUNOSUPPRESSION

P.F. HOYER, G. OFFNER, H.P. KROHN and J. BRODEHL

Department of Pediatric Nephrology, Medical School Hannover, P.O. Box 610180, D-3000 Hannover 61, Federal Republic of Germany

CyA treatment induces a general impairment of the renal function i.e. Inulin and PAH clearances are decreased to the same degree. The nephrotoxic effect is manifest in the early phase after transplantation. Despite the known histological tubular changes associated with CyA nephrotoxicity, no specific influence of CyA on tubular function parameters is demonstrable. During the first year after transplantation GFR impairment is equal in both treatment groups, in the second year we observed a slight further decrease of the GFR. At 1 year after transplantation the GFR correlates with the number of rejection treatments. No correlation was found between GFR and CyA blood levels if blood levels were within the therapeutic range. No CyA induced progressive renal deterioration was found regarding the first and second year after transplantation.

Ciclosporin (CyA) has been shown to be superior to conventional immunosuppression (CIS) after kidney transplantation in children as well as in adults [4,5,6,8]. In our center 2 year survival rates of children and grafts have been 97% under CyA treatment. In contrast; under the conventional immunosuppression with azathioprin and prednisolone the 2 year survival rate of children was 94% and of grafts 68%. However, nephrotoxicity is a considerable disadventage of CyA, leading to limitation of its application. Histologically the nephrotoxicity is visible consisting of tubulo-interstitial alterations like isometric vacuolisation, interstitial cellular infiltrations and fibrosis [1,9]. In the literature evidence for nephrotoxicity is mainly documented by elevated serum creatinine levels. Exact renal function parameters, especially long term side effects in children have not been published. Therefore, kidney function was studied with special emphasis upon tubular parameters.

MATERIALS AND METHODS

The CyA regimen is briefly described (Table I). Starting with 500 mg/m^2/d. In the first week after transplantation, the dosage was weekly reduced until after 5

Correspondence to: P.F. Hoyer, Department of Pediatric Nephrology, Medical School Hannover, P.O. Box 610180, D-3000 Hannover 61, Federal Republic of Germany

TABLE I

Ciclosporin Regimen

Week after tx	CyA (mg/m²/day)	Pred. (mg/m²/day)
1	500 (*)	60
2	450 (*)	30
3	400 (*)	15
4	350 (*)	12
5	300 (*)	9
6	*	6
7	*	4

* Dosage adjustment to blood levels; therapeutic range 200–800 ng/mi.

weeks 300 mg/m^2/d. was reached. Individual dosage adjustments were performed according to CyA whole blood levels [7]. A range between 200 and 800 ng/ml was aimed at as therapeutic level. Prednisolone was started with 60 mg/m^2/d. and was weekly reduced until 4 mg/m^2/d. was reached 7 weeks late

Our experience with this regime is of interest for the farther discussion of the renal function data. The actual CyA doses administered according to this regime are depicted in Fig. 1. The means of the given doses demonstrate the applicability of our regime. The calculated CyA doses in relation to mg/kg/BW revealed higher dose equirements in children when compared to regimes employed in adults (Fig 2).

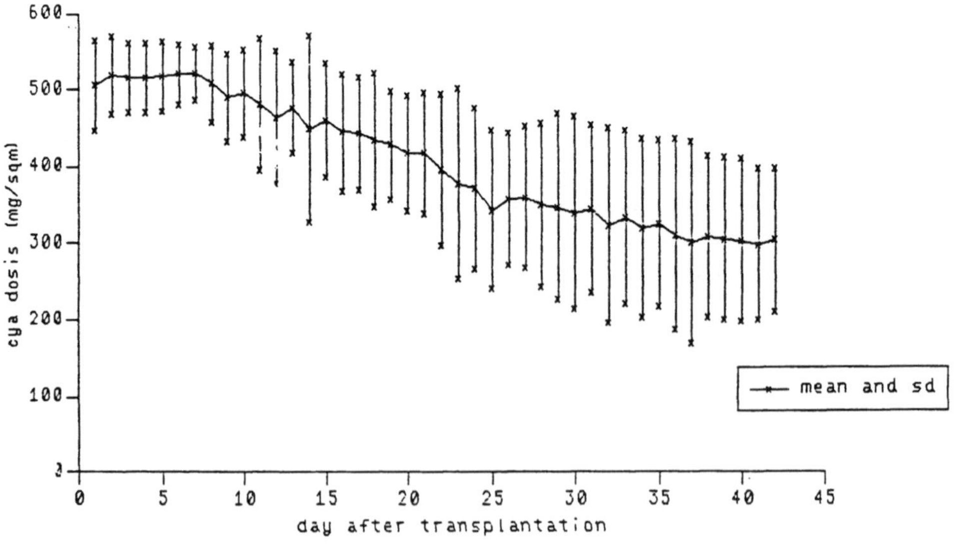

Fig. 1. CyA dosis (mg/m²) after renal transplantation (n = 20 pat.)

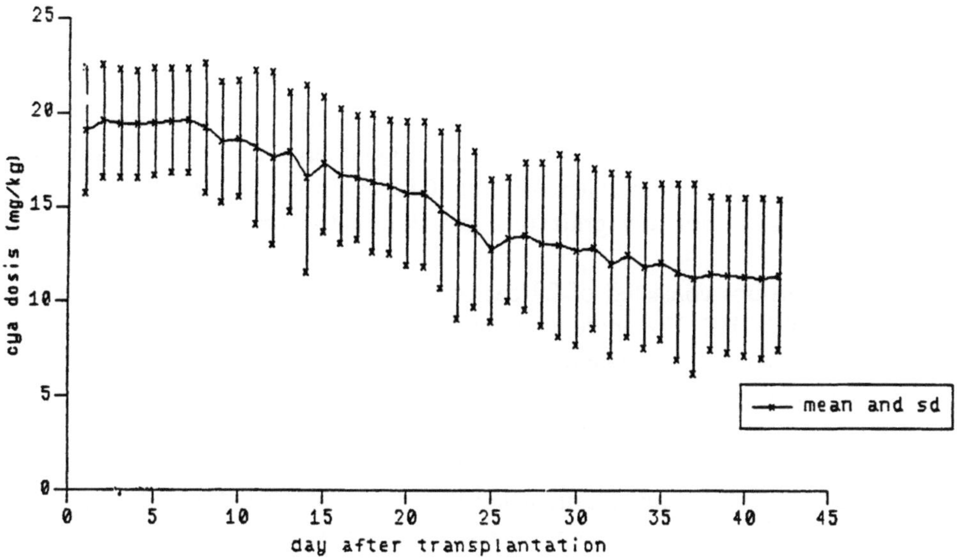

Fig. 2. CyA dosis (mg/kg) after transplantation (n = 20 pat.)

In the second week after transplantation a high variability of CyA levels occurred requiring individual doses adjustments in both directions (Fig 3). From 6 weeks after transplantation it was possible in almost all cases to maintain the levels in the desired range.

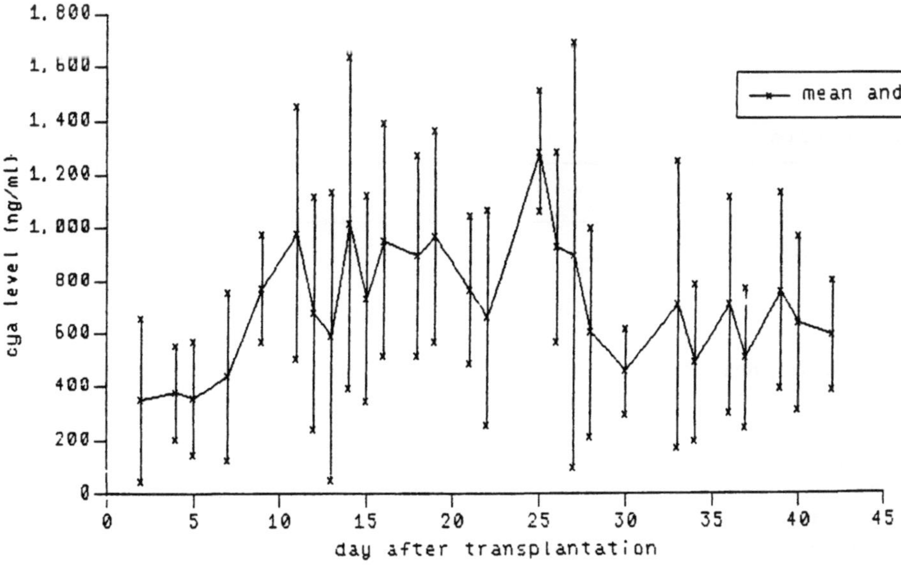

Fig. 3. CyA blood levels after transplantation (RIA).

Renal function parameters of children transplanted between Sept 1982 and Jan 1985 and treated with CyA were compared with those obtained under CIS during the immediate preceeding period from Jan 1980 to Sept 1982. In the latter group, patients with graft loss due to irreversible rejection within the first 2 months after transplantation were not included. In the remaining patients, no further graft losses occurred during the first year. Therefore, the CIS group was comparable with the CyA group, because not any graft was lost during the period covered by this investigation.

The patient groups consisted of 29 patients in the CIS- and 32 patients in the CyA-group (Table II). The male to female ratio and mean age in years were comparable. 26 versus 30 underwent a first transplant, only 3 versus 2 were repeatedly transplanted. The living donor versus cadaver donor graft ratio exhibited more living donor grafts in the conventional group. HLA matches were not statistically different. Cold ischaemia times were comparable. The times required to obtain the lowest (and stable) serum creatinine levels, were equal: 12.3 and 13.9 days.

A higher number of rejection episodes of 1.42 versus 0.88 was encountered in the CIS group after 6 weeks; after 1 year as well as 2 years the numbers were nearly equal (Table III).

Investigated parameters, 6 weeks after transplantation, were Inulin- and PAH-clearance, filtration fraction, fractional phosphate reabsorption and endogenous glucose clearance. At 6 weeks, 1, and 2 years after transplantation serum creatinine and urea. The GFR according to Schwartz et al. [2,3] was calculated from bodylength and serum creatinine, while in addition the calcium and glucose excretion were determined. Statistical analysis was achieved with the T-test, Mann-Whitney U test,

TABLE II

Patient and graft data

	CIS	CyA	p
Number of patients	29	32	
Male/female	14/15	14/18	
Mean age in years	11.8 ± 3.0	12.3 ± 3.5	n.s.
range	7–16	5–16	
Number of transplantation			
1st/2nd/3rd TX	26/3/–	30/–/2	
LD/CAD	14/15	5/27	
B+DR matches	1.95± 0.89	14.1 ± 1.18	n.s.
DR matches	0.95± 0.5	0.84± 0.64	n.s.
Cold ischaemia time	15.9 ±14.3	20.9 ±11.6	n.s.
Day of lowest creat. after transplantation	12.3 ±12	13.9 ±14	n.s.

TABLE III

Number of rejection episodes per patient

	Pat. group	Mean	SD	p
6 weeks after tx				
	CIS	1.42	1.1	
				0.04
	CyA	0.88	0.9	
1 year after tx				
	CIS	2.24	1.7	
				0.43
	CyA	1.87	1.9	
2 years after tx				
	CIS	2.33	1.86	
				0.98
	CyA	2.32	2.26	

Wilcoxon rank est and standard regression using the SPSS X software provided by SPSS Inc.

RESULTS

Serum creatinine levels 6 weeks after transplantation revealed a mean of 78.4 μmol/l $\pm$ 47 for the CIS group and of 103.3 $\pm$ 50 for CyA ($p=0.054$). Consequently CyA nephrotoxicity seems to be not very impressive.

Ranges of Inulin and PAH clearances for the CIS group were mostly within normal limits. In contrast: values in the CyA grou were below the normal limit (Fig. 4).

Six weeks after transplantation Insulin and PAH clearenc s were statistically better in the CIS group than in the CyA group (see Table IV).

Tubular parameters were of special interest because of the predominantly tubulo-interstitial changes seen histologically. Fractional phosphate reabsorptions were not different. The slightly decreased mean for the CyA group is explained by the lower GFR in this group. The glucose clearances were pathologically elevated but here again no difference between the groups is visible (Fig. 5). Glucose and calcium excretion per day, 6 weeks and 1 year after transplantation exhibited equal results in both treatment regimens (Table V,VI). The high amount of glucose excretion in both groups 6 weeks after transplantation, may be explained by the high doses of prednisolone. One year after transplantation the glucose excretion is nearly normal,

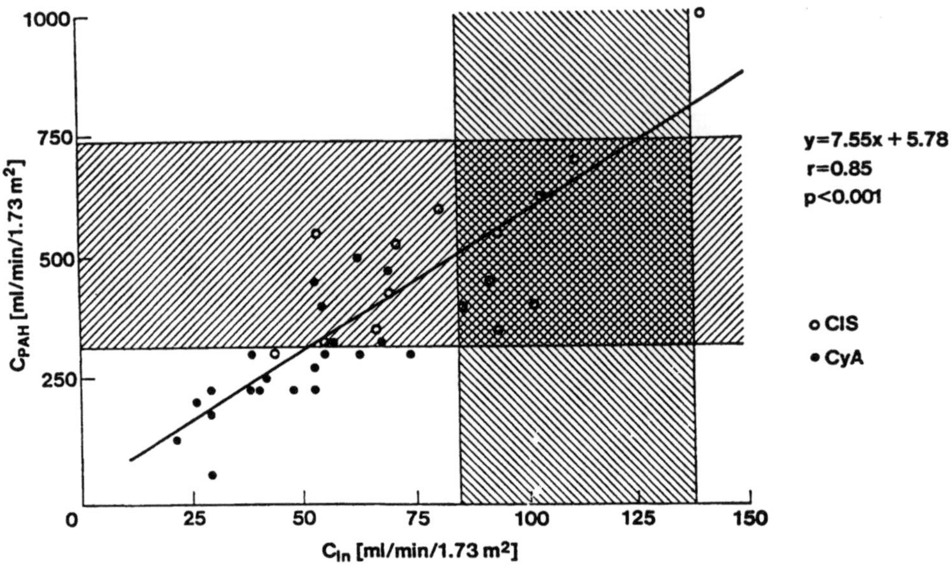

Fig. 4. Inulin and PAH clearance 6 weeks after transplantation.

at this time the prednisolone doses are low in both treatment groups.

The applicability under CyA treatment of the calculated GFR according to Schwartz [10] is demonstrated by its correlation with the measured inulin clearance (r=0,85; see Fig 6).

TABLE IV

Inulin and PAH clearance 6 weeks after transplantation (ml/min/1.73 m²)

	Pat. group	Mean	SD	p
Inulin	CIS	83.16	25.2	0.001
	CyA	47.1	16.4	
PAH	CIS	503.1	181.3	0.002
	CyA	271.0	110.7	
Filtration fraction	CIS	17.1	4.3	0.36
	CyA	19.1	8.6	

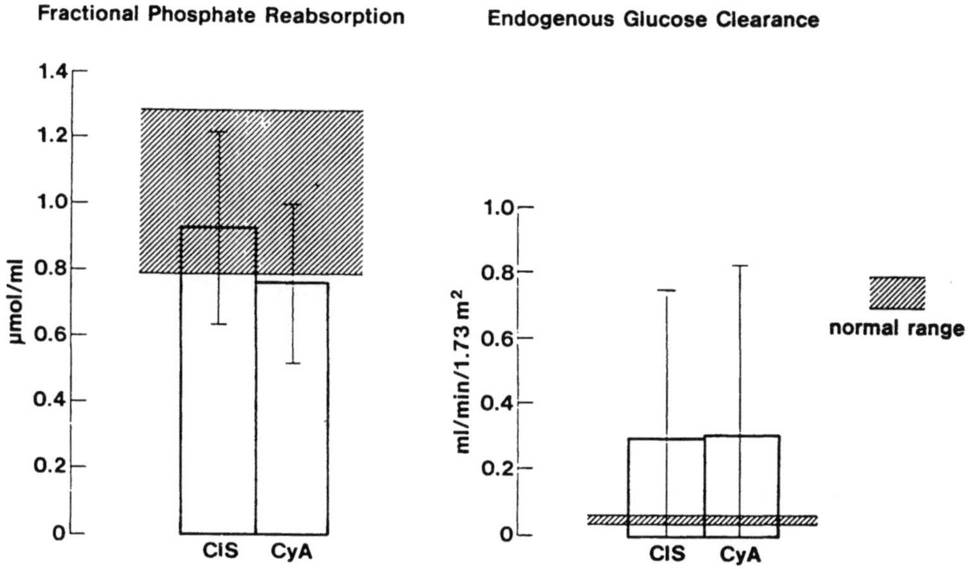

Fig. 5. Clearance data weeks after transplantation.

In the conventional group, the GFR dropped from 80 to 68 ml per min per 1.73 m^2 6 weeks and 1 year after transplantation and 62 ml after 2 years; the correspondent values in the CyA group were from 59 to 46 to 43 (Table VII). Serum urea levels in the 2 groups remained unchanged, but were higher in the CyA group corresponding to the lower GFR. We tried to elucidate the drop of the GFR in the CyA group, because this has not been described in the literature.

TABLE V

Calcium excretion per day
(Normal <0.15 mmol/kg/day)

	Pat. group	Mean	SD	p
6 weeks after tx				
	CIS	0.131	0.07	
				0.99
	CyA	0.137	0.08	
1 year after tx				
	CIS	0.108	006	
				0.32
	CyA	0.099	0.08	

TABLE VI

Glucose excretion per day
(Normal <0.01 mmol/kg/day)

	Pat. group	Median	range	p
6 weeks after tx				
	CIS	0.545	0.302–1.265	
				0.159
	CyA	0.256	0.03 –3.419	
1 year after tx				
	CIS	0.02	0.008–0.104	
				0.129
	CyA	0.016	0.002–0.053	

TABLE VII

GFR SCHWARTZ (ml/min/1.73 m²) at various intervals after transplantation

	Pat. group	Mean	SD	p
6 weeks after tx				
	CIS	80.5	26.3	
				0.001
	CyA	58.9	20.9	
1 year after tx	CIS	68.1	26.9	
				0.001
	CyA	46.4	18.0	
2 years after tx				
	CIS	61.1	25.5	
				0.005
	CyA	42.5	15.8	

The correlation of the CyA blood levels with the GFR is depicted in the scattergram (Fig. 7). Six weeks fter transplantation no relationship is visible and also 1 year after transplantation no dependency can be discerned, when the levels are in the assumed therapeutic range. The GFR 6 weeks after transplantation exhibited no relationship to the number of rejection episodes. However, 1 year after transplantation the GFR correlated inversely with the number of rejection treatments (Fig 8). Therefore, it seems conceivable that one major cause for the GFR impairment during the first year is repeated rejection episodes, similar to conventional treatment.

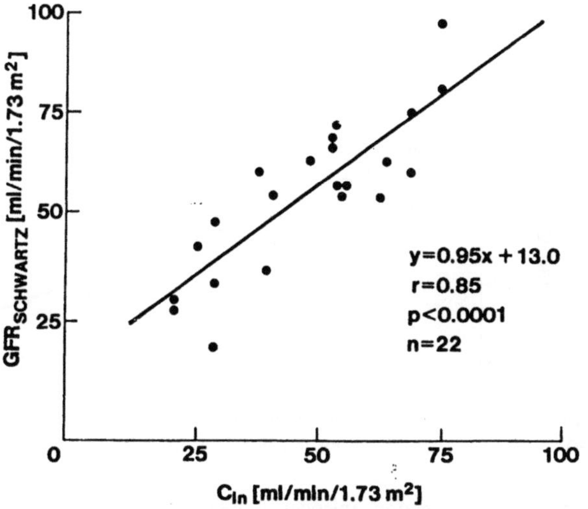

Fig. 6. Correlation between inulin clearance and GFR SCHWARTZ under CyA-treatment.

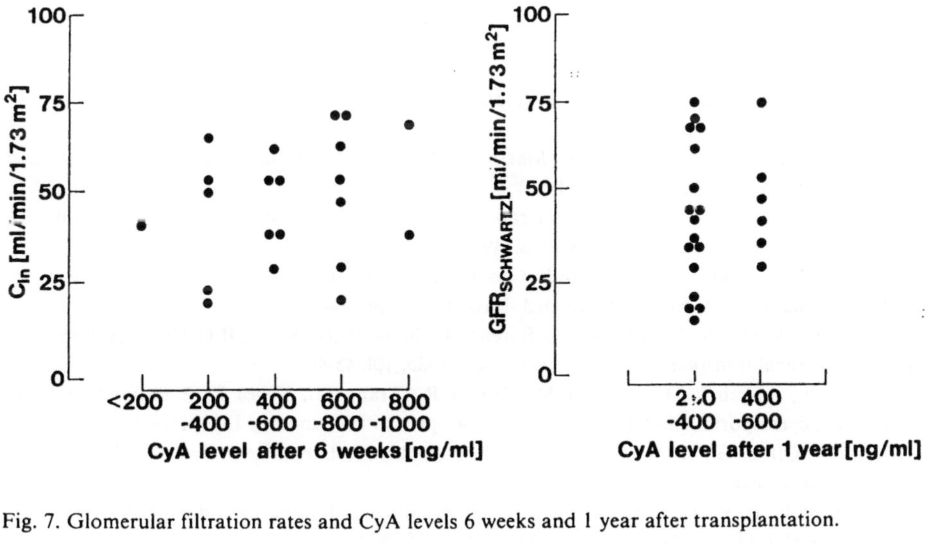

Fig. 7. Glomerular filtration rates and CyA levels 6 weeks and 1 year after transplantation.

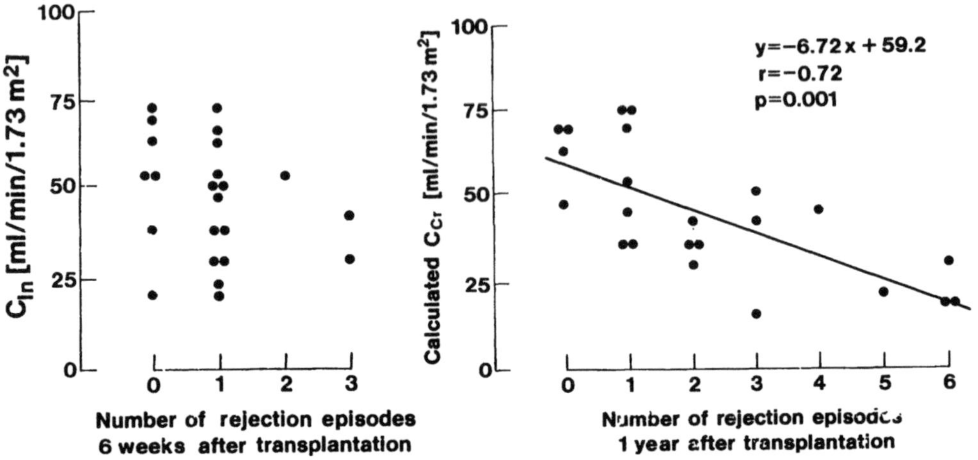

Fig. 8. Glomerular filtration rates and number of rejection episodes 6 weeks and 1 year after transplantation.

REFERENCES

1 Bergstrand A., Bohman S.O., Harnsworth A. et al. Renal histopathology in kidney transplants recipients immunosupressed with cyclosporin A. Clin. Nephrol. 1985; 24:107-119

2 Brodehl J., Gellissen K., Weber H-P. Postnatal development of tubular phosphate reabsorption. Clin. Nephrology 1982; 17:163

3 Brodehl J., Franken A., Gellissen K. Maximal tubular reabsorption of glucose in infants and children. Acta Pediatr. Scand. 1972; 61:413

4 Calne R.Y., Wood A.J. Cyclosporin in cadaveric renal transplantation: 3 year follow up of a European multicentre trial. Lancet 1985, ii:549

5 Canadian Multicenter Transplant Study Group. A randomized clinical trial of cyclosporine in cadaveric renal transplantation. N. Engl. J. Med. 1983. 309:809-815

6 Conley S.B., Flechner S.M., Rose G., Van Buren C.T., Brewer E.D., Kahan B.D. Use of cyclosporine in pediatric renal transplant recipients. J. Pediatr. 1985; 106:45-49

7 Donatsch P., Abisch E., Homberger M., Traber R., Trapp M., Voges R. A radioimmunossay to measure cyclosporin A in plasma and serum samples. J. Immunossay 1981; 2:19-32

8 Hoyer P.F., Offner G., Wonigeit K., Brodehl J., Pichlmayr R. Dosage of cyclosporin A in children with renal transplants. Clin. Nephrol 1984; 22:68-71

9 Mihatsch M.J., Thiel G., Spichtin H.P. et al. Morphological findings in kidney transplants after treatment with cyclosporine. Transplant Proc. 1983; 15:2821

10 Schwartz G J., Haycock G.B., Edelmann C.M. jr., Spitzer A. A simple estimate of glomerular filtration rate in children derived from body length and plasma creatinine. Pediatrics 1976; 58:259–263

OVERVIEW OF THE VARIOUS CICLOSPORIN TREATMENT PROTOCOLS FOR PEDIATRIC RENAL TRANSPLANTATION EMPLOYED BY THE PARTICIPATING CENTERS.

ERIK D. WOLFF[1], ABRAHAM P. PROVOOST[2]

Departments of Pediatrics[1] and Pediatric Surgery[2], Erasmus University, Rotterdam, The Netherlands.

Preparatory to the workshop, questionaires were sent to all participating centers, regarding their CyA treatment schedule, drug monitoring, number of children treated with CyA i.e. for primary or secondary immunosuppression, and the frequency of side effects. All 14 centers returned their questionaires. Approximately 300 children had received CyA as primary immunosuppressive agent, but the 14 treatment schedules differed in detail. However, 5 types of CyA treatment protocols could be distinguished. In 4 schemes CyA was started at the time of transplantation, while in the 5th one CyA was only started after a delay of 1-3 weeks (2 centers). Two centers used CyA only for a time limited period of 3 or 6 months. In contrast, 2 other centers deliberately avoided the use of any other immunosuppressive agent as soon as possible. Six centers used a combination of CyA and steroids. while the last 2 centers used a combination of CyA, steroids, and AZA. All centers monitored CyA drug levels in plasma or blood. Six used plasma or serum, 5 times employing a RIA and one HPLC. Eight used whole blood, 7 times RIA and one HPLC. The desired drug levels ranged from 50-150 ng/ml for plasma RIA and from 150-800 ng/ml for blood RIA. No clear conclusions could be drawn from the questionaires concerning the side effects of CyA in children after renal transplantation or the impact of the various treatment schedules on the side effects. Detailed information is provided by the contributions of the various centers to this book.

Preparatory to the Workshop questionaires were sent to the various participating centers (Table I).

In this questionaire we asked for information concerning the use of ciclosporin (CyA) in pediatric kidney tranplantation. Although all questionaires were completed, it was not easy to draw firm conclusions from the answers. We were able to compare the various treatment schedules and the therapeutic monitoring of the CyA levels during treatment. For details about the various side-effects of CyA the reader is referred to the individual contributions of the Workshop participants.

Correspondence to: E.D. Wolff, Nephrology division, Sophia Children's Hospital, Gordelweg 160, 3038 GE Rotterdam, The Netherlands

TABLE I

CENTERS PARTICIPATING IN THE WORKSHOP:
"CICLOSPORIN IN PEDIATRIC RENAL TRANSPLANTATION"

CITY	COUNTRY	CLINIC	PARTICIPANT
BERN	(SWI)	UNIV. CHILDRENS HOSP.	O.H. OETLIKER
BRUSSELS-1	(BEL)	CLIN. UNIV. ST. LUC	Y. PIRSON
BRUSSELS-2	(BEL)	HOPITAL BRUGMANN	F. JANSSEN
ESSEN	(FRG)	UNIV. KINDERKLINIK	K. PISTOR
HANNOVER	(FRG)	MEDICAL SCHOOL	G. OFFNER/P.F. HOYER
HEIDELBERG	(FRG)	UNIV. KINDERKLINIK	K. SCHAERER
HOUSTON	(USA)	UNIV. TEXAS MED. SCH.	S.M. FLECHNER
LONDON-1	(UK)	GUY'S HOSPITAL	G.B. HAYCOCK/S. RIGDEN
LONDON-2	(UK)	ROYAL FREE HOSPITAL	R. TROMPETER
MUNICH	(FRG)	KLIN. GROSSHADERN	B. KLARE
NEW YORK	(USA)	DOWNSTATE MED. CTR.	A. TEJANI
NIJMEGEN	(NETH)	RADBOUD HOSPITAL	M. DE JONG
PARIS	(FRA)	HOP. ENF.-MALADES	M.F. GAGNADOUX
TORONTO	(CAN)	HOSP. SICK CHILDREN	D.F. GEARY

CICLOSPORIN TREATMENT SCHEDULES

The schedules employed by the various centers all differed in detail. However, five main protocols could be distinguished shown in Table II. Two centers employed a CyA treatment schedule (A) aimed at the early withdrawal of other immunosuppressive drugs. In six centers CyA was used in combination with prednisolone only (B). Two centers used the triple combination of CyA, prednisolone and azathioprine (AZA) (C), whil two other centers used the same triple combination, but deliberately postprotocols after administration of CyA by 1 week (Toronto) or 3 weeks (Paris) (D). range the initial period antilymphocyte globulin was used. In 2 centers CyA was only used for a fixed period (E), amounting to 3 months in Nijmegen and 6 months in London-1. In London-1, prednisolone and AZA were used in combination with CyA. In Nijmegen CyA was given in combination with prednisolone and replaced by AZA.

CICLOSPORIN MONITORING

In all 14 centers CyA levels were monitored in blood or plasma to adjust the daily dose. As indicated in Table III, 6 centers used plasma or serum while 8 centers used whole blood. A radio-immunoassay, usually measuring CyA plus an unknown amount of metabolites, was applied in 12 centers, while HPLC, measuring CyA only, was applied in 2 centers.

TABLE II

CICLOSPORIN TREATMENT SCHEDULES FOR PRIMARY USE IN PEDIATRIC RENAL TRANSPLANTATION

A	CyA	--	MUNICH
	PRED	--	NEW YORK
	AZA		
B	CyA	--	BERN
	PRED	--	BRUSSELS-2
			ESSEN
			HANNOVER
			HEIDELBERG
			HOUSTON
C	CyA	--	BRUSSELS-1
	PRED	--	LONDON-2
	AZA		
D	CyA	------------------------------------	PARIS
	PRED	--	TORONTO
	AZA		
	ALG		
E	CyA	--	LONDON-1
	PRED		
	AZA		
	CyA	--	NIJMEGEN
	PRED		
	AZA		

CyA = CICLOSPORIN
PRED = PREDNISOLONE
AZA = AZATHIOPRINE
ALG = ANTI LYMPHOCYTE GLOBULIN
--- = INDICATOR OF THE DURATION OF DIVERSE MEDICATION

CICLOSPORIN SIDE-EFFECTS

As in adult renal transplant recipients, the most frequent side effects of CyA were: nephrotoxicity, hypertension, hypertrichosis, tremor and gingival hyperplasia. Because of the relatively small numbers of children in each of the various treatment

TABLE III

DESIRED CICLOSPORIN TROUGH LEVELS DURING TREATMENT

PLASMA/SERUM		BLOOD	
	RIA (ng/ml)		RIA (ng/ml)
BRUSSELS-1:	<100–500	BERN:	400–800, later 150–400
BRUSSELS-2:	50–150	ESSEN:	400–600
		HANNOVER:	250–750
HOUSTON:	50–100	HEIDELBERG:	200–400
		LONDON-1:	400, later 300
PARIS:	50–120	MUNICH:	300
TORONTO:	<100	NIJMEGEN:	400–800
	HPLC (ng/ml)		HPLC (ng/ml)
LONDON-2:	50–150	NEW YORK:	100–200

schedules, no clear conclusions could be drawn about any divergence of the frequency and severity of side-effects between the various combinations.

PROPOSAL FOR FUTURE EVALUATION OF CICLOSPORIN TREATMENT SCHEDULES IN PEDIATRIC RENAL TRANSPLANTATION.

There is no consensus regarding an optimal immunosupressive treament schedule after kidney transplantation in children. Consequently, each center developed their own particular schedule aimed at maximal patient and graft survival with the largest possible reduction in number and severity of side effects. Five main schedules could be distinguished for CyA treatment. However, no conclusions could be drawn from the information supplied in the questionnaires or from the individual contributions regarding transplant survival or effective reduction in the number and severity of side effects. Most centers, including those transplanting 50 children per year will need at least 4 years before any conclusion can be drawn comparing two diverse treatment schedules. We therefore propose an International Coöperative Study which, albeit cumbersome, might reveal "more definite" answers in a shorter period of time. The centers participating in the workshop have responded positively promising to coöperate with such an international working group. We sincerely hope that this will enable future evaluation of different CyA treatment strategies in pediatric renal transplantation in an efficient and definitive manner.

Bei Fragen zur Produktsicherheit wenden Sie sich bitte an:
If you have any questions regarding product safety,
please contact:

Walter de Gruyter GmbH
Genthiner Straße 13
10785 Berlin
productsafety@degruyterbrill.com